DIETING IS AN ABSOLUTELY PERSONAL EXPERIENCE!

Depending on how much weight you want to lose, how fast you want to lose it, and—just as important—the personality traits you bring to any diet, one or two plans will be most effective for you. Remember that the same diets may be totally unworkable for your best friend. The trick is to sort through all the diets to find the one that will fit your needs.

That is what I will help you do with my book.

—Corinne T. Netzer

THE
RIGHT
DIET BOOK

How to Really
Lose Weight

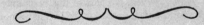

CORINNE T. NETZER

A DELL BOOK

To Evonne Rae

Published by
Dell Publishing Co., Inc.
1 Dag Hammarskjold Plaza
New York, New York 10017

Dell ® TM 681510, Dell Publishing Co., Inc.

ISBN: 0-440-14667-4

Printed in the United States of America
First printing—February 1977

Illustrations by Giorgetta McRee

"He who does not mind his belly
will hardly mind anything else."

—Dr. Samuel Johnson

CONTENTS

FOREWORD:
A WEIGHTY PROBLEM

I am a great believer in last flings. Before getting married, before starting a new job, before you go finally and irrevocably broke; in fact, before you do just about anything that requires buttoning down in some new way—and that includes dieting. So, as a personal favor to me would you, right now, put down this book, march yourself to the refrigerator or cupboard or wherever you keep your private stash of fattening rewards and have a ball! Stuff your stomach, eat yourself silly! Indulge your particular food passion, whatever it happens to be, until all you can do is smirk. Do it, whether it takes a quart of butter rum ice cream, a whole Sara Lee chocolate cake, a pound of spaghetti drenched in butter or a double bag of bet-you-can't-eat-just-one chips (my own weaknesses, every one). Keep on eating till you can't anymore. I want you to have an orgy with gusto. Without hesitations. Without guilt. And without a thought to your weight.

Dieting is serious, but the most serious requirement for losing weight is maintaining your sense of humor, right? So consider this your last fling, your one last great self-indulgent blast before beginning our all-out war on your waistline.

Ready, set, enjoy!

O.K. Now that you're feeling contented, we can get down to business. You know the problem, I know the problem; every month an estimated 10 million of us try to cope with the problem: Food Glorious Food, or How to Keep Your Shape in Shape in This Land of Too Much Plenty. It isn't easy when food happens to be our national pastime. Eating is bona fide entertainment, one of the ways we Americans best enjoy ourselves. When we entertain at home, we proudly offer our friends great quantities of specially prepared food, and when our friends reciprocate, it's usually for brunch or dinner. An evening on the town is likely to center on a good restaurant, afternoons spent with the kids more often than not wind up at McDonald's, and major family occasions are more often than not celebrated as 15-course feasts.

If you spend any time thinking about it, you'll probably realize that a good number of your waking hours are occupied with food. If you're not actually eating then you're buying food, planning to buy it, preparing it, even fretting over its prices. It's hard for any but the most iron-willed soul to escape the national food obsession. Food, when you come right down to it, is even the method we use for telling time: breakfast, mid-morning coffee break, lunch, mid-afternoon snack, late afternoon nibble, dinner, after-dinner treat, before-bedtime snack. Who needs clocks anymore?

It's no wonder that between 75 and 100 million Americans are overweight, and unhappy about it. Every woman's magazine regularly features a "spectacular, all-new" diet, which, according to sales experts, is a major factor in these magazines' consistent success. And our leading newspapers continue to herald innovative diets or announce diet scandals week after week. Second only to stories about Jackie Onassis, dieting articles are the papers' most popular drawing cards.

Yes, we're all too aware that we're too fat. But why are 58% of us tipping the scales well over our normal weights? Why haven't we yet stopped ourselves from overeating?

As a perennial dieter who has been poring over diet books and articles for over 15 years, I don't think there's a single theory that has escaped my fanatic eye. Which to believe? Well, over the years, I've concocted a personal theory about my own weight problem, borrowing a fact or an intuition when they apply to me. I'd suggest you do the same for yourself, and to start you off, I'll give you a rundown of the major schools of diet thought.

Getting down to basics is the way some scientists examine the overweight problem, and "basics" means your genes. According to this school, if Mama is warm and loving and generous and also very large, and if Poppa is jovial, fun-loving and fat, there's an 80% chance that you will inherit their tendency to overweight. It just runs in the family, say the scientists. Hope, however, resides with those choosing to dismiss this rather fatalistic theory; after all, it has never been conclusively proved.

In the sociological camp, obesity is blamed on eating patterns developed during childhood. The fault, these experts claim, lies not in our traits, but in our training. My cousin Dodie, 32, who weighs in at a substantial 150, 25 pounds over her desired weight, has only recently remembered that from the time she was old enough to use a knife and fork, her mother, my aunt, hefted gargantuan portions of food on her plate at every meal. After she had cleaned her plate, there were always seconds, whether she was full or not. All her life, Dodie has eaten this way without even considering the existence of another method of dealing with food. A perfect example of the "bad habits" school of diet theory, Dodie was trained from infancy to believe that overeating is normal.

Parents lay the groundwork for the eating patterns which each of us carries into adulthood. From our mothers, we learn the types of food we prefer, the amount we consume, and when and why we eat. Unfortunately, this early training can lead to our forming bad habits, which are psychologically difficult for an adult to break. In addition, overeating during the early years of life appears to increase permanently the number of fat cells in our bodies. The more fat cells you contain, the closer you'll have to watch your weight—forever. You don't necessarily have to be fat, but to prevent it, you will always have to be extra prudent.

About 20 years ago, experiments performed with laboratory rats produced a brand-new theory of overweight. Not only did it cause a general hullabaloo, but it also served to vindicate millions of overweight Americans who could now claim, "It's not my fault! There's something wrong with my system!" These lab studies focused on the hypothalamus, the tiny control center in the brain which regulates our appetites or our desire for food. When the scientists deactivated the hypothalamus in rats, the animals went berserk. They ate compulsively and constantly, never able to satisfy themselves. Applying reverse logic, the theorists posited that, if hypothalamus abnormalities did indeed cause obesity, then obesity was probably caused by this physiological disturbance! While the theory for a short time absolved a lot of overeaters of personal responsibility, it was later demonstrated that very few humans actually suffer from this malfunction.

You may already be familiar with hypoglycemia, or low blood sugar, because it's one of the primary points of Dr. Robert Atkins' theory of overweight. Dr. Atkins, along with other authorities in the field, contend that hypoglycemia is responsible for obesity in vast numbers of Americans, and that by controlling a person's blood sugar level, we can begin to control his weight. When the body is low in blood sugar, a substance which fuels the brain and nerve tissues, distress signals are sent out to the brain: more glucose! more glucose! The person experiencing this distress develops a craving for carbohydrates, the foods which the body immediately converts to glucose. Consistently low blood sugar causes an almost continuous desire for high-carbohydrate foods such as candy, cake, ice cream, potatoes and pasta. Almost without exception, high-carbohydrate foods are super-fattening when consumed in generous quantities, and so, the person gets fat. And fatter. Again, turning this cause-effect relationship around, this school points out that overweight people *do* crave carbohydrates—so they are probably hypoglycemic! The theory, however, does have a number of important detractors who have been quick to point out that the symptoms of hypoglycemia—rapid pulse, perspiration, feelings of shakiness or dizziness—are identical to symptoms brought about by plain and simple anxiety, and that it's anxiety, not hypoglycemia, which causes many people to overeat carbohydrates. Personally, I can identify with this situation, since my first instinct in a stress situation is to head straight for the refrigerator. The test for hypoglycemia is a simple one that can be performed in a doctor's office, so if you're suspicious of your blood sugar level because of any of the above symptoms, I'd recommend making an appointment to have the hypoglycemia test.

So far we have no clearcut answers to the question we first asked: why are so many of us so fat? If we can't find an honest scapegoat in our genes or in our body parts, where *can* we lay the blame?

I've read about loads of terribly ingenious obesity experiments done with fat people in controlled laboratory situations. Although the data are ultimately inconclusive, it really is fascinating.

- Obese people do not know when they are hungry.
- Obese people do not know when they are full.
- Obese people eat more than "normal" people in stress or fear situations.
- Obese people eat by the clock; that is, when they are "supposed" to be hungry.
- Obese people eat in relation to the availability of food.
- Obese people eat in relation to the taste of food—more of a good-tasting food.
- Obese people rarely commit suicide.

Hardly a reason to overeat, but there you have it.

For me, the obesity theory that carries the most weight concerns itself with our national food habits. Which brings me back to my initial point of food as an American preoccupation. The American lifestyle is fast and busy, which means cooking shortcuts and meals on the run. The advent of fast-food chains, as well as the explosion of junk and frozen foods, may be easier on our schedules, but they're murder on our hips and thighs.

Let me tell you a story. Arline, who is one of my oldest and dearest friends, recently called me up one evening in a panic. She had treated herself to an evening of beauty, according to the advice of some article she'd been reading in a leading fashion magazine—luxurious, perfume-scented bath, shampoo and hair conditioning, leg waxing, skin creaming, manicure, pedicure, the works. She felt exhilarated and more relaxed than she'd felt in weeks; that is, until she set her newly-polished toes on the bathroom scale. Clean-scrubbed, rose-scented and sexy, she weighed seven pounds more that what she'd weighed two weeks before! Why, she wailed, as if I had the magic answer (I have to tell you that as a kind of lay diet expert, my overweight friends are constantly calling me with unanswerable questions like this). I told her that I honestly couldn't say off-hand, but to take heart; we'd soon identify the problem. With Holmeslike accuracy, I narrowed the field until, interrogating Arline about possible changes in her eating habits, she timidly offered that she'd been having lunch every day—for the past two weeks—at the new fast burger joint that had just opened up down the block from her office.

Giant double cheeseburger, French fries, fruit pie and a strawberry shake. Well, that'll do it every time. (The story has a happy ending. Arline, for the next two weeks, remained glued to her desk every noon with cottage cheese and a banana—her own private crash—and managed to take off each last shake-induced pound.)

And Arline isn't unique.

Are you getting the picture? It's no wonder we're a nation of chronic fatties!

Food has also become chic. I personally have more friends who can whip up a quick *ragout de boeuf borde-laise* than can cook a simple, old-fashioned pot roast. They all seem to be enrolled in exotic cooking courses. French, Chinese, Indian . . . It's divine for me as an enthusiastic dinner guest, but I can't tell you what it's doing to their waistlines, which seem to expand with their gourmet repertoire. Eating gourmet-style, which means eating expensively (just price out those esoteric ingredients) is emblematic, and like a second car or a swimming pool, another sign of our conspicuous consumption. Isn't it true that eating expensively means you've "made it"?

Second cars. That brings up another important point. You probably feel as guilty as I do about not getting enough exercise, which we all know is the super shaper-upper. I'll have to admit that it's a rare day when I'll spend the extra half-hour or 45 minutes it takes to walk if I can get there by car, bus, subway or train in 10 minutes. Like everyone else, my inner clock is geared to a fast pace—get there, get it done and get on to the next activity. Unfortunately, little of all this frenzy is actually physical—my perspiration index is set at practically zero, my most strenuous activity being pencil pushing and typing. Yes, I try to remember to do a few deep knee bends and sit-ups every morning, but calisthenics was never my thing, and most a.m.'s I'm dressed and out the door before remembering that I've forgotten to do them! While tennis and skiing are enjoying new and well-deserved popularity with a lot of folks these days, most Americans are still participating in the sport that exercises only part of the body—the eyeball.

We're all aware that the time we spend in front of the TV is time that could be better spent in some more active and beneficial (to our figures, anyway) form of recreation. We watch our favorite TV performers knocking themselves out dancing, singing or chasing the bad guys while we loll in our chairs, stuffing ourselves with junk food. Or we sit immobile in front of the set, hypnotized by the Superbowl or the World Series, and actually work up enough of a thirst to polish off several calorie-filled colas during the game.

Again, echoes can be heard from millions of overweights across the country: "But nobody ever taught me *which* foods were fattening!" There is a great deal of truth in this line of defense. As a nation, we are grossly ignorant in the areas of health and nutrition. Most of us have no idea how our bodies function. And we couldn't really describe what good health is all about. Aside from those nutrition charts that used to be pinned up in our grade-school classrooms (remember the four basic food groups?) and the one week the home economics teacher devoted to "our bodies" (for girls only), Americans receive *no education at all* in these areas. But that's not really surprising. Our own government has thus far exhibited little concern in the overall health and well-being of its citizens; our medical schools are appallingly negligent in teaching future doctors about nutrition; nor has television been a crusader in this important field. Personally, I would like to see the TV networks offering prime-time weekly programming in health, nutrition and physical fitness, special shows for children as well as for adults. So much of what we learn comes via this influential medium that I believe television has a responsibility to educate the public in these crucial areas.

Well, off the soapbox.

I must be making you just a little bit impatient. When, you probably want to know, is she going to tell me how to fit into that bikini I wore last summer? Or that dress, now two sizes too small, that I want to wear to my friend's wedding? Where's the magic formula that's going to get those awful pounds *off*?

The magic formula doesn't exist. The only answer, as you well know, is to diet. Diet, diet, diet, diet. Say it over and over again, because you and I are going to have to get good and used to the idea of doing without all those fattening foods we've come to adore. There's simply not another way to lose weight.

Men and women have been formally dieting for over a hundred years. At a time when Americans were deep into the strife of our own bloody Civil War, the very first diet book was being published in England, at the personal expense of a rich London coffin-maker who magnanimously wanted to share with other obese Victorians the wondersome diet that had caused him to lose nearly 50 of his 202 pounds—in one short year! Overweight must have been a household word for them, because the first 1000 copies of William Banting's pamphlet *Corpulence* proved so enormously popular that Banting published a second edition just a year later, and once again the copies became coveted properties among the plump dowagers and parliamentarians of London. You may be surprised, as I was, to learn that Banting's wonder diet, created for him by physician William Harvey, was a plain and simple low-carbohydrate regimen that restricted carbohydrate intake to just 60 grams per day!

Well, they say there's nothing new under the sun, and it's true that every single low-carbohydrate or high-protein diet since that first one has been just a chip off the old Banting. Vilhjalmur Stefansson's *Eskimo Diet,* a big splash in the 1930s; the *Holiday Diet,* created for overweight executives of the DuPont Corporation and popularized by *Holiday* magazine in 1950; the controversial *Calories Don't Count* diet to which millions subscribed in the early sixties; the inimitable Dr. Irwin Stillman's *Quick Weight-loss Diet,* famous for its eight sloshing glasses of water a day; and most recently, Dr. Robert Atkins' *Diet Revolution,* first billed as the "*Vogue* Super Diet," are all part of the same big diet family. Each and every one of these diets operates on precisely the same principle: that if you restrict the intake of carbohydrates, the body is forced to use its own stored-up fat as a source of energy.

Here's the essence of low-carbohydrate dieting: depending on the particular diet plan, the dieter partakes of from 0 to 60 carbohydrate grams daily. More than this amount of carbohydrates is considered by theoreticians to be superfluous—and fat-producing. From Banting on down, the low-carbo people have rallied 'round the slogan, "We're fat because we eat *the wrong foods.*" These "bad foods" are considered to be high in carbohydrates. Even more recently, the accusing finger has been pointed by this camp at certain specific offenders—refined white sugar, bleached white flour and hydrogenated fats, all of which Americans consume in overwhelming quantities. Nutritious proteins and fats, insist Stillman, Atkins et al., are generally healthier foods, since the human body is able to utilize them more completely than carbohydrates.

The second school of dieters doesn't count grams at all; instead, they count calories, a calorie being a measure of the amount of "energy" value contained in food. I don't think there's anyone who isn't acquainted with low-calorie dieting. Its banner slogan shouts out, "We're fat because we eat *too much!*" In low-calorie diets, you simply cut down on what you eat. It's quantity that's important here, and so, under this broad umbrella, come diets as wildly different as the essentially conservative Weight Watchers program and the radical Cottage Cheese Crash. Just how much you cut down is the crucial thing; what you eliminate from your diet determines how fast you'll drop those extra pounds.

Low-calorie dieting also has a past, and like low-carbo dieting, its history begins in 19th-century England with a restrictive diet devised for the portly King George IV by his personal physician, a stern gentleman (and I would guess, thin himself) who lacked Mr. Banting's sympathy for the overindulgent and underexercised. At about the same time, another London doctor was recording the very first "crash" diet in which he recommended a rather meager fare of lean meat and stale sea biscuits(!) for a retired butcher who adopted it, apparently with satisfactory results.

But we were dieting in America, too. Across the ocean, the first water diet splashed into the news. Advertised by a New York socialite, Celia Logan Connelly, who, like so many of us, had run from diet to diet without being able to lose any of her excess poundage, Dr. J. H. Salisbury's special reducing system had at last enabled her to lose 30 pounds in six months! The diet was essentially a low-calorie regimen. It also prescribed that the dieter "quench the thirst by drinking, about one hour before meals and retiring, all the water that the body craves—drink nothing else between meals."

We continued to "cut down" for a decade, but it wasn't until 1911, when the *Journal of the American Medical Association* published the very first calorie chart, that we actually started counting calories to lose weight. From then on, dieting was strictly a numbers game.

In the Roaring Twenties, Dr. Lulu Hunt Peters decreed 1200 calories a day for safe weight loss. In the 1930s the magic number was 1500, the count urged by Chicago Health Commissioner Dr. Herman Bundessen for overweight Americans. As a nation, we didn't diet during the war years, but nutritionists, the new scientists, impressed upon us the importance of eating "balanced meals" and this philosophy carried over into the Eisenhower era when Harvard University, foremost in nutrition research, came out with their *1400-Calories-5-Meals-A-Day Snack Diet,* a sane program for inveterate nibblers.

Those dime store calorie counters became the dieter's best friend, helping her through the U.S.D.A.'s *Uncle Sam Diet,* the 1200-calorie *Grapefruit Diet* and most recently, Jean Nidetch's *Weight Watchers*—low-calorie diets, each and every one.

Low-calorie dieting has the power of the establishment behind it; so far, it's been the method preferred by nutritionists, and certain plans have also been endorsed by the American Medical Association and various public health groups. If you've dabbled at all in diet literature, you're probably aware of the continuing battle between advocates of low-calorie dieting and the proponents of the low-carbohydrate method of weight loss—it's been going on for as long as I can remember. Furious charges have been hurled by each group at the other. Each claims that the other is nutritionally unsound. Each claims that the other is leading dieters down the rosy road to high cholesterol levels, high blood pressure and heart disease. Even charges of political self-interest have been mentioned as reason for preferring one diet method over the other.

Let me state right here that I don't endorse one diet or diet system above another. As a dieter, not a doctor or nutritionist, my purpose is not to decide an argument which has been raging for years, confounding even the experts. What I have learned, from personal experience, is which particular diets work for *me* and what the best way is for *me* to lose weight.

Dieting is an absolutely personal experience. Depending on how much weight you want to lose, how fast you want to lose it and the personality traits you bring to any diet, one or two or possibly three plans will be the most effective ones for you. Remember that the same diets may be totally unworkable for your best friend. The trick is to sort through all the diets to find the ones that meet your own needs.

What I will say on behalf of all the diets I describe, whether low-carbohydrate or low-calorie in philosophy, is that they all work. And they have worked for millions of reducers over the years.

INTRODUCTION:
FOOD FOR THOUGHT

My sole purpose in writing this book is to help you to lose weight. Whether it's a quick five pounds that have to be taken off before next weekend, or a cumbersome 30 that you're finally getting around to tackling, you should be able to find some helpful information, guidance and possibly encouragement in the material I've gathered here. As I mentioned before, I've been reading diet books and magazine articles for years. Some of this material I've found to be pure nonsense. A lot of information, on the other hand, is worthwhile and valuable for people like us to know. What I've done here is to sort through volumes of material (believe me, there are volumes) in an effort to separate the wheat from the chaff.

Anyone who is or has ever been overweight knows that fat is not fun. Personally, there is nothing that makes me feel more insecure than walking into a roomful of people when I know that my dress is one size too small or that I've got a range of brand new dimples where I never had any before.

We all have the potential to look better and feel better and, who knows, if you've never been at your desired weight before, finding that diet which works for you may open up whole new worlds. Sometimes a change in your self-image is all it takes.

I am not out to convert you. There isn't one particular diet that I endorse above another. The right diet, as far as I'm concerned is the one that works for *you,* the diet that's going to whisk away those unwanted pounds. You won't find me trying to persuade you to do things *my* way. I won't try to change your life-style to fit some eating scheme that's incompatible with your real habits and personality.

There are enough diets in this book—so that after reading through them, you'll probably be able to pick out three or four that you like well enough to try. Let me warn you that the first diet you attempt may not be the plan you finally end up following. For one reason or another—either the types of foods included, the quantity of food allowed, the number of times you're allowed to eat or the too-high cost of the plan—the first diet you launch may be all wrong for you. Don't be discouraged. Simply pick another diet and try *it* out. If the same thing happens, try a third plan. My friend Leslie went through four—the Cottage Cheese Blitz, the Grapefruit Diet, the 5-Day Diet, and Dr. Atkins' Diet—before finally losing 12 pounds on the Eat-to-Lose-Weight Diet, a more gradual regime that fit her temperament perfectly. I will say that if, after five or six tries, you *still* haven't found a diet you can stick to, it may be time to examine whether you're really serious about losing weight. You may just be inventing excuses to keep from facing the problem.

I've also tried to make this book a kind of primer on diets, health (as it relates to diet) and nutrition. By the time you finish reading it, I hope you'll have a general picture of how the body utilizes food, the general nature of different foods and what quantities of food your own body requires for optimum health. At the risk of sermonizing, I'll repeat that health is one of the big reasons for losing weight, as important or more important than looking thin.

The material I've included is organized so as to be readily accessible, to enable you to find the information you need without too much groping around. The following chapter answers the question: how fat is "fat"? And while it may sound like a silly question with an all-too-obvious answer ("you're fat if you look fat or feel fat"), there are doctor's definitions for overweight that every dieter should be familiar with, as well as a list of sound medical reasons for losing weight, as if you needed that kind of prodding. At any rate, I believe this information is as valuable as the actual diets themselves.

Next, a chapter explaining how we become overweight; that is, why you woke up one morning and couldn't fit into your favorite skirt or pants suit. And if you still don't know what a calorie is, though I can't believe there's an American who doesn't, you'll find the whole story on chemical shifts and balances there, too. I have a lot of friends who keep talking about slow metabolisms, which they pinpoint as the reason for their overweight. Frankly, it's easy blame in a lot of cases, but if you believe you're one of life's "slow burners," the information on body metabolisms—and your physician—will help you to bear it out.

I know that while it's interesting to discover how weight goes on, the reason you're reading this book is to find out how it comes off and to find a diet that will work for you where others have failed. What makes one particular diet more successful than another is covered in my chapter on the psychology of dieting. Dieting is more than simply sticking to the rules. Losing weight involves a change of mind, literally, and a drastic shift in the way we think about food and eating. Old habits, like dashing for the icebox every time you become anxious, or overeating whenever you visit your parents, are so ingrained and so much a part of all of us that unless you're aware of them, these devils will do a good job of subverting your best diet intentions. So I've put together a do-it-yourself therapy manual for would-be dieters, gleaned from my own experience and from friends' successes and backslides. Also, this chapter will lead you to the diet that's best suited to your life-style, personality, eating habits and budget, as well as your timetable.

Then come the diets themselves. I'll say now, and repeat again later, that's it's important to consult your physician before embarking on any new diet. While there's nothing intrinsically dangerous about losing weight, it is a good idea to have your physician pronounce you in good health before you begin. If you're rundown, or otherwise ill, a postponement may be suggested, and it's wise to follow your physician's advice in this case. The doctor who knows your medical history may also have special reasons for preferring that you follow a particular weight-loss program. Again, do as he or she says.

When you get the go-ahead, you should read through all the diets before choosing one. While some of the plans may be familiar because of the tremendous amount of publicity they've received, others you've perhaps never heard of might better suit you. Also, getting acquainted with the whole gamut will give you a pretty accurate picture of the world of dieting—what the fuss is all about.

I've started out with *the low-calorie plans,* which have long been favorites of people who don't like a radical change in their eating habits and who need the strict limitations imposed by counting calories. Skim through these. One of them may be right if your big problem in losing weight is willpower.

The low-carbohydrate diets, contrarily, seem to be extremely effective for people who have other problems. Do you put on weight after just a single slice of cake or plateful of pasta? Low-carbo dieting may be your best answer to weight control, since it cuts your intake of fat-producing carbohydrates to the barest minimum. Or if you've had repeated failures with low-cal regimens, the complete turnabout in eating habits dictated by most low-carbohydrate diets may provide the novelty that other diets lack. Another big advantage: on low-carbo diets, you won't suffer those gnawing hunger pangs that can foil the most determined among us; since you're allowed virtually unlimited quantities of "stick-to-the-ribs" proteins and fats, your stomach is always satisfied. Still another plus is that you don't have to count *everything*—you only keep tabs on carbohydrate grams, and many foods contain no carbohydrate grams at all.

Next are *the crash plans,* those out-and-out frontal assaults on fat. Most of us have crashed at some point, so you probably know what a lifesaver the right crash diet can be in a real crisis; for example, when you have to lose five pounds by the end of the week to fit into your only black cocktail dress. These ultra-low-calorie diets will trim flab off quicker than you can say "cottage cheese, please," and there's a crash for every set of taste buds. Whether your own particular fondness is for strawberries or hot dogs, farm-fresh eggs or packaged bologna, you can build a workable diet around that food. Since it's the only thing you'll be eating all week, these one-item diets have the added advantage of being ultra-cheap—if a bit monotonous. Crash diets, let me point out, are not recommended for anyone with health problems. And no one, not even those in tip-top condition, should stay on a crash for any longer than one week.

The only diet that gives more dramatic results than crash dieting is really a no-plan diet, or more accurately, *a no-eat diet: fasting.* Again, while fasting is definitely not prescribed for anyone but the super-healthy—and your physician will best determine if you are—a two or three day program of near-abstinence (on most fasts you're allowed unlimited liquids as well as vitamin-mineral supplements) is sometimes a marvelous way to begin losing weight, especially for those who have a long, long way to go. That initial five-pound weight loss may provide a bounty of encouragement, and enough incentive to resolve you stick to the regular diet plan you've chosen. See my special section on fasting for specific how-to's.

There are some folks who will wash out of any diet plan after a few days. The truth is that some people just cannot diet for love nor money. It's simply beyond their natures. If you're that type, the answer to your weight problem might be *a group-action program* like Weight Watchers, Overeaters Anonymous or TOPS. Peer support, encouragement and even chastisement when you've broken the rules are often enough to motivate even the most recalcitrant dieter. I've devoted a chapter to the various organized group plans in existence or, if you prefer dieting in the company of good friends, there are suggestions for forming your own neighborhood group. Check this section if you're a "people person"— with a fat problem.

I close this chapter with a round-up of *my own diets,* inventions I've worked out over the years to deal with a seesawing weight problem. Again, I stress that I'm not commending these to you, since some may be too peculiar for anyone but me. It's just possible, though, that one of them may strike your fancy, and I can guarantee that all of them work. I also guarantee that you won't find these diets in any other book in the world! In this chapter you'll also find a collection of "forbidden food substitutes," tried-and-tested low-carbohydrate recipes for the breads, cookies, candies and other fattening goodies that most carbo-counting dieters sorely miss.

By that point, you'll probably have picked out a diet you can live with and, as I've said already, this diet will fall into one of two categories: it will be either low-calorie or low-carbohydrate. The following big section is crucial to your success or failure. To enable you to follow your regimen without buying another book, I have included a complete calorie, protein, fat and carbohydrate gram counter. Over 1500 common and uncommon foods are listed here, each one given in everyday household measures. Whether you're counting calories or grams, keeping track of proteins or watching your intake of fat, you'll want to refer to this guide on a daily basis.

The last chapters complete your diet education. Don't skip the section on nutrition, at least not if you want to maintain your beautiful new figure forever. Everything you'll need to know about *devising a lifetime maintenance plan* is contained here, including a chart of the whole alphabet of essential vitamins and minerals needed for good health. Since exercise figures in most diet plans, I've included simple bend-and-stretch routines perfect for toning up those tired old muscles as you're trimming your weight. If you don't get regular physical activity, like walking, biking, jogging, swimming or tennis, consider a program to start off each day.

Generally speaking, I balk at advice given by "experts," but I'm especially sensitive when it comes to losing weight. Doctors, nutritionists, Ph.D.'s in physiology or biology—granted, these knowledgeable people often have valuable information to impart, and they frequently even have our best interests at heart, but . . . we fatties are a sensitive bunch, and we're unusually suspicious of anyone who hasn't been through it himself. The immediate reaction to lecturing, scolding and other efforts at re-education is likely to be a defensive "what do *they* know about being heavy, anyway?" That's also why advice from skinny friends is particularly hard to take.

Only another overweight person knows how it feels to look in the mirror and suddenly realize that your image is much larger than you ever thought *you* were. Or how it feels to say you haven't got a thing to wear, and really be telling the truth. Or what it means to fail at one diet after another after another. Or finally to succeed in losing your excess weight only to gain it all back again, each and every last pound.

I am not a diet doctor. I am not a nutritionist, nor do I have advanced degrees in any field of science. I am a dieter. What I've learned about losing weight over the years has been through personal experience and lots of reading, from which I've drawn conclusions about my own weight problem. I won't pretend that what has worked for me will necessarily work for you. Each of us has a unique body chemistry, which, combined with a unique personality and unique way of living, makes rules about losing weight impossible. Besides, letting you do things your own way is only democratic, right?

Where I can, I will pass along to you some things I've learned. For example, plus and minus points for various diets; hints, tricks and tips to make any diet more effective; experiences I've had with different plans and diet stories that friends have repeated to me; and the encouragement that every would-be thinnie craves when faced with a bleak week, or two weeks or month of doing without one of life's great pleasures: food. The rest, dear dieter, is up to you.

HOW FAT IS "FAT"?

How do you know when you're fat? Most people simply know, that's all. When I lived in Florida, I had a neighbor whose constant complaint was her weight, although to my eyes she was attractive and slim enough in her tropical size nine fashions. One day, after not seeing her for several weeks, I ran into Rosalie in the supermarket. She looked different, and much better, though I couldn't put my finger on the change. What was it? Despite everyone telling her that she was neurotic, Rosalie had gone on Dr. Stillman's Quick Weight-loss Diet and had lost seven pounds—the seven that made the difference between looking good and looking great. She *knew* she was fat, even if no one else thought so.

Whether you're petite or large-boned, short or tall, lean or muscular, you're a candidate for overweight—anybody can get fat. Knowing that doesn't solve any immediate problems, but there is some perverse satisfaction (it's there in all of us) in knowing that it can happen to anyone. Being overweight makes you neither ill nor unique.

I've been bandying this term "overweight" around, so you should probably know how it's properly defined and how it's different from that other nasty word, "obesity." Start with these notions: (1) An obese person is not always overweight; nor is an overweight person always obese, and (2) being overweight is not always bad; being obese, on the other hand, is never good! Sound like double talk?

Overweight, according to the experts, means you weigh more than you *should* weigh according to the norms of sex, age, height and body type. In *pounds,* you're over the limit. Obese means that your body is carrying too much fat—more than the 15% of total body weight considered normal and healthy by the experts. When a person is obese, he or she is over the limit in *fat*.

I hope you got that: normal and healthy. Fat is good. Fat is not a dirty word. Be assured that every human being needs to carry some fat on his or her body for normal functioning. Not only does fatty tissue act as our natural cushioning and insulation, but it's also the body's own storehouse of energy. If, for example, you were stranded on a desert island for three days without food, your body would burn its own fat for fuel, and providing you had water, you could easily survive.

As I said, 15% of the body's total weight is all the fat you should be carrying around. With more than that, you're in the category of obesity. How does that happen? Food is energy. When all the food you consume is burned up by the body in its normal activities, your weight remains constant, and so does your body fat. In other words, you use up everything you intake in a lovely, balanced flow of energy. But suppose a person does *not* burn up all the food he or she has eaten. When that happens, the excess is stored by the body, usually in the form of fatty tissue—those rolls, lumps, bulges and bumps we're all too familiar with. (This equation of food intake and energy expenditure is measured in terms of the calorie, a handy calculating unit I'll tell you more about in the following chapter.)

Are you thinking now that maybe you are obese? Well, technically it may be true, but kindness commonly calls the condition overweight—obese is a little harsh on us poor overindulgers. But back to my riddle. How can an obese person not be overweight, and why is someone who's overweight not always obese?

The answer lies in those "norms" that tell us what we are *supposed* to weigh, according to statistics. These statistics, most of them compiled by our nation's insurance companies, are based on large population samplings. They indicate average weights for Americans based on sex, age, height and body type. Thus, if you are a woman who is five feet five inches tall with a medium frame, the "Desirable Weight Chart" (see p. 44) puts you between 110–122 pounds. That's what most women with your body type weigh. For most people, the charts are useful as a general guide, but, as with everything else, exceptions to the rule do exist.

Here's one snag; let's hypothesize two women, both five feet five inches tall and both with a medium body build. Call the first Marie, and the second Sandy. Marie works as a secretary. She holds a regular 9 to 5 job, and for relaxation on the weekends she likes reading, going to plays and movies and doing needlepoint projects which she sells to a local boutique. Her life is interesting, but as she admits, it's pretty sedentary. Not much exercise, though she's forever meaning to join a health club. Sandy, on the other hand, is super-active. During the week, she works as a tennis instructor at the Y, and on Saturday and Sunday loves nothing better than to go backpacking in the mountains with friends. She's a mover, going all the time.

Marie weighs 120 pounds, within the "desirable" range for her height and body type. But she is flabby and she feels fat, the result of not exercising enough. On the other hand, Sandy hasn't weighed 122, the upper limit of the "desirable" range, in years. For her, the scales balance at 125, but she's never felt better in her life. Lean and muscular, she's in superb condition.

Yet, according to the charts, Sandy is overweight and Marie is not. See how misleading statistics can be? In truth, there's no reason in the world for Sandy to lose weight so long as she's healthy and feels and looks attractive. Marie, however, probably should go on a diet or, better yet, start exercising to convert some of her flab to muscle. As far as obesity goes, Sandy would not be considered obese, while Marie, whose body fat is more than 15% of her total weight, *is* obese. Get the point? So, rely on the charts as a general indicator, but do consider the "fat factor" before branding yourself overweight.

How much fat is too much fat? And how can a person tell when the percentages start creeping up beyond 15%? While you could check in at the local hospital for the "soft x-ray" test that films your fat tissue to get an answer, there are three other good tests to determine whether or not you're too fat, and they can all be done within the privacy of your own home.

Mirror, mirror on the wall . . . one of the unavoidable facts of life stares us directly in the eye when we take the ruthless mirror test. I would suggest you do this one when you're alone. Strip down and stand in front of a (non-distorting) full-length mirror. Do you like what you see? Is the reflection of your nude body pleasing to you? Now jump up and down. Are the jiggles the ones that are natural? Or is the movement being made by layers of fat shifting position? Hard as the looking glass is, it gives the most honest answer about overweight.

The second test is known as the "pinch and feel" test. In children and in adults through middle age, fat is stored in the subcutaneous tissue layers just beneath the surface of the skin (in elderly people, fat may go deeper), and so fat may be gauged by an outward measurement. Experts have determined that the normal amount of fat should go no deeper than one-half inch beneath the epidermal layer; more than one-half inch signals too much fat. Take the "pinch and feel" test this way: using your thumb and forefinger, grasp a fold of skin at some place where you suspect fat, like your waist, belly, thighs, hips, derriere, calves, upper arms or upper back (you'll need some help for that last one). If the fold is more than one inch in thickness—remember, a fold is two layers of skin added together—it's time to find yourself a good diet. If the fold is under one inch thick, you're doing fine. Do check at several different spots, though, since people are quirky about how they gain weight. While your midriff may remain trim, fat-prone hips could be doing a wild spread all of their own accord.

The ruler test diagnoses abdominal fat, or as it's commonly known, the spare tire. Use a regular school ruler for this. Again disrobed, lie flat on your back with your legs close together. Place one end of the ruler on your ribcage and the other end on your pubic bone. If the ruler touches both, consider yourself home-free. If the ruler can't touch both bones, but wobbles around on the mound of fat that's between them, you're a candidate for one of the diets in this book. The ruler doesn't lie!

O.K. Now you know it for sure. You're fat and something must be done about it. As if you didn't know already, but . . . how much weight should you lose? What is your ideal weight?

Five or six pounds put on over the holidays or while you were on vacation is simply a matter of resolution. You know where you stand and what you have to do. Depending on what kind of diet you choose, you can get back to your normal weight in one or two weeks with relatively little anguish. I know, because I've done it dozens of times.

It's just possible, perhaps probable, that you've been carrying your excess baggage around for so long that you no longer have any idea what "normal" is for you. Do consult the "Desirable Weight Chart" on page 44. As I said before, this chart should be used as a guide *only;* it is not the final word by any means. See if the weight listed for your height and body build sounds right; if it does, gauge your weight loss by that number.

A still better guide is your past weight. Most of us can remember a time when we felt great and felt we looked great. For me, it was between the ages of 21 and 24, when I was an eager young girl with her first big job in the big city—with all that running around, meeting new people and dancing till the wee hours in New York's raucous discotheques, there was no time to eat! If you can recall your thinnest year, you'll know your ideal weight—the weight at which you were attractive, physically fit and terrifically confident. Use this standard for planning your diet. Another useful control comes from the insurance companies, which provide us with so many statistics about ourselves. In agreement with many medical authorities, they claim that our ideal weight is what we weighed during our early twenties. So, if you weren't overweight at 21 or 22, consider this figure.

For individuals who *have* been overweight since high school or since childhood—and there are lots of folks who have—I would strongly urge that you consult your doctor before taking another step. For two good reasons: first, you probably have no idea what your ideal weight is; and second, after a thorough physical examination, your doctor may want to put you on a medical diet under his personal supervision. Remember, your problem has been one of a lifetime, so it deserves special attention.

Onward. Armed with your magic number—five pounds, ten pounds, twenty or forty pounds to lose— you're finally on your way to a new Raquel Welch style figure! You've decided once and for all that those awful pounds are going to come off, this time forever. At this point, you should prepare to experience something called wavering resolve. Symptoms? Your intentions start turning to jelly. You begin to consider that there are worse things in the world than being fat. You start thinking of yourself as an all-embracing earth-mother type. Forget it. Vacillation is perfectly normal, so don't be too angry with yourself. After all, you do have a long way to go, and sometimes it can seem pretty hopeless. Here, for morale-boosters, are some good reasons to stick with it.

Carrying around too much weight just feels bad. It's the feeling of being so firmly moored to the ground that the idea of walking to the corner store for a container of milk leaves you winded. It's a heavy sluggishness that goes right down to your very bones themselves. There are some good reasons for it. Too much body fat literally saps your energy. Avoirdupois has increased, but the size of your internal organs hasn't. Heart, lungs, kidneys, liver—they're all exactly the same size as before, only now they must labor more to maintain your extra weight. The result is that overweight people tire easily and feel exhausted much of the time. Health hazards aside, I think you'll probably agree with me that it's simply frustrating not to be able to do everything you want to do because of fatigue.

I'll be hard-hearted about this one. Fat is ugly. I've never seen ripples, rolls or folds that I considered cute or otherwise appealing—on myself or anyone else. Perhaps in foreign cultures where the fattest man is the richest and lives in the biggest house, more is better, but in America we praise an aristocracy of the svelte and the sleek. A trim figure indicates that you care about yourself and encourages other people to care about you, too. As the old saw goes, if you don't, why should anybody else?

From the kitchen to the bedroom. For many overweights, sex is a distressing problem. More than one of my friends has confessed a total lack of interest in love-making or even in close physical contact when she is fat, and I can understand that. Sexy women have a healthy pride in their bodies. If you're embarrassed to be seen naked, chances are your partner is going to feel embarrassed, too. These kinds of vibrations are contagious. Such a situation sometimes has an unfortunate snowball effect, creating real unhappiness within a relationship. I call it the "if-you-don't-love-me-when-I'm-fat-you-don't-really-love-me-at-all" syndrome. Testing a partner in this way spells danger, and playing this game is nothing so much as asking for rejection. You're looking for someone else to blame for uncomfortable feelings you have about yourself. Whatever insecurities and fears you may have, it's likely that they have nothing to do with your partner—they're your own. If this pattern rings a bell with you, even the slightest tinkle, it might be a good idea to discuss the whole thing with your mate. Instead of making him into the enemy, make him aware of your feelings and fears. Someone who genuinely cares about you will want you to be slim. Not for his "love object," but for your happiness.

What else? Well, I know that when I'm at my best weight, people tell me that I'm more fun to be around, more vivacious, and I notice the same thing about them. Feeling attractive is a natural high and a real confidence-booster. When I look good, surprising things happen: I become more articulate, I think more clearly and I'm able to tackle many more challenging situations. For one thing, I'm not constantly preoccupied with my weight and my appearance. Worrying about your fat really takes up a lot of time, not to mention mental energy. With some people, this can reach obsessive proportions. We all know them. They're the ones whose conversation pivots around their weight problem and the current miracle diet that's going to cure them forever. They are unbearably dull—and they never do seem to lose the weight.

Women, take heed! This confidence, this "I'm the greatest" attitude is a super plus point on the job market. It's a fact that women are holding more and better jobs every year, and we're going to continue doing so. Earning money, and earning as much money as possible, is not a luxury anymore. It's a necessity for most of us—for single women who are supporting themselves; for married women whose income is as crucial to the household budget as their husbands'; and for the many women who, as heads of households, are carrying the burden alone. We're out there in full force, and in the business world—the great "out there"—first impressions matter as much as a college diploma. Looks definitely count. In a competition where other qualifications are equal, an employer will generally hire a slim person over someone who is overweight. Sexist, you cry? Not true. The same preference hires trim men over obese. Employers want people who are going to present an attractive, positive image of their company. And, motivated by pure selfishness, they also want people who are concerned about their health and fitness; these people have a proven lower rate of absenteeism. So, why enter the job market with a handicap? Or if you're already working, why hamper your chances for advancing all the way to the top?

Whether you're working for a livelihood or working in the home (that other full-time job), money is always a pressure. Making ends meet is difficult for all but the privileged few. Have you considered that losing weight is a way to trim costs and save up to several hundred dollars every year? This may sound like a sales pitch, but you really can economize by eliminating those quantities of junk foods which are so terribly expensive—empty calories with a sky-high price tag. You may never cut out your junk passion (martyrs *are* dull), but just cutting down can mean the difference that buys a new dress, curtains for the living room or membership in the local tennis club.

Lest these reasons not be enough for you, the medical profession has its own tote sheet of statistics on overweight. The numbers are sobering indeed, but they do add up to one unavoidable conclusion: being fat is hazardous to your health. A few pounds over the line isn't going to kill you, but even simple overweight does multiply the risks and leaves you far more susceptible to certain medical problems than non-overweights. Much as we'd like to ignore them, I think we must consider the facts.

Chronic overweight has been positively linked to heart disease, and heart disease, I'm sorry to report, is still on the upswing in this country. Fatty deposits, because they narrow the arterial passages, slow the natural flow of blood to all our vital organs—heart, brain, kidneys and so on. Thus undernourished, these organs function at less than maximum efficiency. All this can go on for a long time without anyone being the wiser, and that's why being overweight is sometimes called the "silent killer." But should the arteries leading to the heart become *too* narrow because of built-up fat, an individual may suffer a heart attack. If the affected artery is one that leads to the brain, a stroke may occur. The outlook for heart attack and stroke victims is pretty poor; these illnesses are fatal in 50% of cases. And, if men have been the main victims up to now, evidence shows that women are catching up fast. That's not what liberation is all about.

Like cigarette smoking, overweight may wait to show its effects until a person is much older. Many doctors now feel that senility is not a normal function of old age, as it was once thought to be, but rather the result of impaired circulation to the brain due to creeping atherosclerosis—again, those fatty deposits that slow up the blood flow. And if the specter of cardiovascular disease doesn't scare you—it does me—here are some other statistics: your chances of surviving gall bladder disease, cerebral hemorrhage, kidney and liver ailments and diabetes are significantly decreased if you are fat. For women, pregnancy and delivery tend to be much more difficult, and in some few cases fatal, for the obese individual. Finally, the last word from the nation's insurance companies: statistics show that people of normal weight live longer than people who are overweight.

So, there's every reason in the world for you to lose

those extra pounds and no good reason not to. If you've ever been thin before or if you've never been thin before, know that the rewards of dieting are many, not only in terms of how others view you, but in how you feel about yourself. For some, the change in self-image is so positive that it's like the beginning of a whole new life.

HOW WEIGHT GOES ON

Food, glorious food. Food is at the center of a world rich in meaning, calling to mind in all of us a treasury of images and associations. Food, for me, is the supermarket, itself a kind of gastronomical theater for the American shopper, wondrous in imagined possibilities. Food is photos in *Family Circle, Good Housekeeping* and *Woman's Day:* savory stews, chilly California salads and frothy desserts in sparkling custard glasses, all beckoning the reader to test her talents in ever more challenging ways. As an addicted bedtime cookbook reader, I have my food heroes and heroines, too, as you probably do: Betty Crocker, Fannie Farmer, James Beard, Julia Child—their recipes read like intriguing short stories with predictably happy endings. Food also reminds me of people, relatives and friends I've known over the years who are tied in my memory to their particular "special dish." My grandmother to her incomparable sweet and sour pot roast; my mother to cakes, pies and fresh homemade bread; an aunt who cooks Russian-style to sweet beet soup and paper-thin blinis; even my father to hearty breakfasts which are family institutions.

There's none of us who can't tap a well of these savory associations. But while lazily pleasant, the fact that food is so overladen with meaning makes it infinitely more difficult to give up, especially for overeaters. It's also why we often don't see food for what it really is. Stripped of meaning and romance, food is quite simply nourishment for the body, the essential fuel that keeps us alive and functioning.

Eating the right foods will also help to keep you thin. Like different grades of fuel, foods vary enormously. A sirloin steak is as removed from a banana as a head of lettuce is from a loaf of bread. And not just in appearance and taste. Each food has its own private mix of chemical ingredients. What food is made of determines how it's going to be used by your body and, more importantly for you now, whether it's likely to end up as ugly fat tissue on hips, arms and midriff. Some foods spell instant fat; others aren't allowed to progress that far in the body.

Knowing which foods you can eat to your heart's content and which are more expensive in terms of your figure is a must for the serious dieter. Faithfulness to Dr. Stillman or Dr. Atkins or to Jean Nidetch is only half the battle. Of course, you can and will drop pounds on any diet if you eat exactly what's allowed and avoid what's not. The problems, however, arise after you've achieved your weight goal. Maintaining that slender new shape when you're not adhering to a strict regimen is tricky unless you're familiar with certain ground rules that apply to every eating situation.

I assure you that the basic facts about food are easy. Everybody already knows a little something about food, if only that bread exemplifies carbohydrate grams and a big, juicy steak is an example of protein. Or that overeating high-calorie foods is bad. Going a few steps beyond that should be interesting. After all, you're not learning unrelated facts. Since "you are what you eat," it's extra self-knowledge that you're gaining—and that can't be bad.

Here, then, a Crash Course in Food, for all of us who've ever mouthed that dangerous slogan: "I don't know much about it, but I do know what I like."

The food we eat comes from plants and animals, which are living (organic) substances. It's easy to forget sometimes that succotash grows in garden rows as lima beans and corn. The common denominator for all living things, whether plant or animal, consists of certain chemical elements which form the basis of life.

What are nutrients? They're substances which nourish. They sustain life and promote growth. We need nutrients in order to live—as children, for growth; and as adults, to maintain health. Proteins, carbohydrates and

fats help do those jobs for us. Everpresent in the food
we eat, these nutrients show up in changing proportions.
Certain foods contain more of one than another. In
popular shorthand, we call foods carbohydrates, fats, or
proteins, depending on which nutrient is the primary
one in a particular food.

Protein is contained in large quantities in animal
meat, poultry, fish, eggs, nuts, dairy products and some
grains. *Carbohydrates*—sugars and starches—are the
primary nutrient found in fruits, some vegetables,
breads and flour products. *Fats* are abundant in milk
products, oils, meat, nuts, dairy products and certain
grains.

Nature, being economical as well as efficient, assigns
to each of these three food nutrients a different function
in the body. Protein, carbohydrates and fats each do a
specific job.

Of the three, protein is the hero. Protein comes from
the Greek word *protos,* meaning first, and this complex
nutrient really is most important. For this reason: protein contains essential substances called amino acids,
sometimes referred to as the body's "building blocks."
When you eat any food containing protein, secretions in
your stomach go immediately to work on it, forcing the
protein to release its valuable amino acids. These are
then able to get on with their own work: amino acids
are assimilated by the body's cells for the crucial tasks
of growth, upkeep and repair of organs, blood manufacture, maintenance of the hair and skin and formation of
disease-fighting antibodies.

If protein is responsible for the basic nature of your
body's cells, carbohydrates are the activating power for
these cells. This is the nutrient that pushes your brain to
think and your muscles to move. Carbohydrates are
super-fast workers. They are converted by the body to a
simple sugar for instant energy; anything you don't need
right away is efficiently stored as another sugar, in the
liver and muscles. Or, it's converted directly to fat for
storage.

Fats, too, are energy, but the long-term brand. Fat
does other important work in the body (it forms cell
membrane materials and helps to absorb vitamins and

cholesterol) but fat's most serious job is to be housed by the body as a source of fuel. Stored in fat cells, fat is ready energy when you need it.

All this activity goes on silently and efficiently, without your even being aware of it. How the body converts food into usable substances is true cause for wonder. This network of processes, all going on simultaneously, produces the energy that sustains your life.

Energy. Hard to understand, harder to describe. Think of it as a kind of power, a vital force. Energy is being created and used all the time. It's created by the body utilizing food, and used up by the body for all its activities in a natural, continuous cycle. Difficult to measure, energy is described by scientists in terms of a more understandable unit, the calorie. The calorie simply measures heat, the heat released when energy is used or produced. Measure the heat and you know how much energy there is.

What does all this have to do with losing weight? Plenty. As you know, food is measured in calories. All that means is that different foods supply your body with different amounts of energy. A slice of white bread gives 62 calories, a 4 ounce hamburger supplies 326 calories, a 12 ounce glass of beer is 151 calories, an average banana is about 100 calories. Energy values, all.

Now, on the balance side, your body *requires* a certain number of calories to function. Some calories are for involuntary processes like keeping your heart pumping, lungs expanding and body temperature normal. Other calories are for everything else you do, from waving your arm or chewing your food to sprinting a record-breaking mile. In an ideal world, the number of calories you take in equals the number of calories your body needs. Calories in = calories out. Energy in = energy out. That's a system where all things balance perfectly. And where your weight remains stable.

But shift the balance to one side or the other, and your weight seesaws, too. Pounds are gained when you intake more calories than you use up, and vice versa. What's happened is that you've produced more energy than you need, and the body's only recourse is to store it up for the future—as fat.

Who hasn't counted calories? Anyone who's ever been overweight knows the nitpickiness of monitoring each last daily morsel, each tidbit that passes one's lips. Low-cal diets restrict the number of calories you eat to fewer than the amount you actually need to function. Now your body is forced to mobilize its stored fat. Called into action, old fat is burned to make up the energy difference. So, you lose weight. Depending on how drastically you cut calories, you'll drop fat slower or quicker.

The process isn't all that mysterious. In fact, weight loss is accurately figured by referring to two standards: first, the total number of calories that you, as an individual, require; and, second, the number of calories that creates a pound of fat.

Scientists have calculated that one pound of body fat is worth 3500 calories. Overeat 3500 above what your body needs, and you've gained a pound. Slice 3500 from your diet and watch that same pound melt away. It's a fixed equation. Your caloric needs are a bit harder to figure; the number is individually determined by adding the calories needed for daily activities to the calories your body burns when at rest (known as your basal metabolism rate). Since individual needs differ based on sex, age and body size, and vary, too, because some people are more active than others, charts have been devised to make it all a bit easier. Do consult the "Caloric Maintenance Chart" on page 159 for your own caloric requirements.

A general rule of thumb in figuring your caloric needs is to multiply your "desirable weight" by 15 if you are a pretty sedentary person, or by 20 if you're very active. (Most of us, I'm afraid, fall into the sedentary category!) The number you come up with is the number of calories you should eat every day if you want your weight to remain stable. When you diet down to normal weight, this will be your magic number: don't consume any more calories if you don't want to gain! Consult your doctor to see if he agrees with this daily calorie requirement for your own particular needs.

Cutting calories makes pounds disappear, and I'll get into the specifics of low-cal dieting a little later on. What kinds of foods you eat isn't important, so long as you keep within your calorie limit. Then watch your weight go down, down, down.

If you're wondering what proteins, carbohydrates and fats have to do with the price of ice, they add some interest to the calorie story. They're leading players in the drama since they determine the caloric content of a food. Fat provides your body with the most energy: each gram of fat supplies 9.3 calories. Proteins and carbohydrates each give 4 calories per gram energy value. Apparent, isn't it, why fats go straight to your hips? They're high-calorie storable energy. But what about carbohydrates? They certainly don't deserve a "bad guy" reputation when protein has the same calorie value!

A fascinating point, and the rationale behind all low-carbohydrate and high-protein dieting. Though identical in energy values, these two nutrients are in other ways vastly dissimilar. (1) Carbohydrates are easily stored. Protein is not. Liver, muscles, and fat cells welcome excess carbohydrates; contrarily, the body utilizes protein down to the last bit. (2) It takes *five times* as much energy for the body to burn protein as it does carbohydrates. That means you use up five times more calories digesting a lamb chop than digesting a baked potato.

Overeating is the only reason most of us are fat; don't let anyone try to convince you otherwise. We're unhappy about our figures because we've stockpiled them with an arsenal of unusable calories. Fat is food, and too much of it. To be perfectly fair, though, other factors can sometimes influence weight and cause us to balloon out without apparent cause. These are most often disturbances of the glandular system. Rare occurrences to be sure, they can cause weight gain.

You've heard people refer to a "thyroid problem." The thyroid is just one gland in the body's intricate endocrine system. Endocrine glands secrete hormones, which act as instigators and regulators of normal bodily functions. The thyroid is the gland that controls metabolism, the rate at which you burn your food and convert it to energy. This is done by means of a secretion called thyroxin. If the thyroid is off kilter, too much or too little thyroxin is manufactured. An abundance causes rapid burning of food, but when too little thyroxin is made, metabolism grows sluggish. (Remember my friend with the slow metabolism?) Many experts discount thyroid disturbance as the sole cause of obesity, but if you have reason to suspect a deeper reason for your own problem, mention it to the physician at your pre-diet examination. A thyroid test will evaluate its capacities.

In the first chapter, I mentioned hypoglycemia. There's been a lot of hooha about it lately, and many people who aren't hypoglycemic are convinced they are. Hypoglycemia is low blood sugar, which means too little glucose (sugar) in the blood. Blood sugar is regulated by insulin, a hormone secreted by the pancreas. Underproduction of insulin causes diabetes, high blood sugar, while an oversupply causes the body to burn sugar too fast, resulting in depleted supplies for the brain, nerves and muscles. Symptoms of hypoglycemia are hunger, faintness, perspiration, shakiness, anxiety—and a distinct craving for carbohydrates, which are the foods that give relief. Hypoglycemia, however, is not all that common—certainly not rampant, as a few experts have suggested. Again, the majority of us are overweight because we overeat. Check with your doctor about hypoglycemia if you commonly experience those symptoms listed. It's just possible, though unlikely, that you've got low blood sugar.

Diseases associated with other glands (sex glands, hypothalamus and pituitary glands specifically) can result in obesity, too, but in these instances an abnormal distribution of fat may be apparent, not just simple fat. And because of other, more serious effects, you and your doctor would be well aware of that kind of condition. Hypochondriacs, relax.

In passing, one more villain in overweight: prescription medications. Some are fat-producing. Birth control pills, for instance, seem to promote water retention in women, which appears on the body as fat. If you are taking regular prescription drugs and are experiencing a simultaneous increase in weight, it's probably a good idea to check in with your doctor. He'll be able to advise you best.

Knowing how you put on those extra pounds is helpful—you'll know how *not* to repeat the mistake. But what you need to do right now is to get those pounds off, fast. Finding the diet that's going to trim you, slim you and turn you into the very attractive person you really are underneath it all is next on the agenda—you're halfway home already.

DETERMINING YOUR DIET PLAN

Losing weight is easy once you've made up your mind to. Actually, the decision to go ahead with it is probably the most difficult part of anyone's diet, since fat is a problem most overweights have been living with, worrying about and procrastinating over for years. Dieting means a kind of coming to grips with the awful truth and for most, blessed relief. When you get right down to it, taking full responsibility for yourself feels pretty good.

You should give yourself a pat on the back for getting over the biggest hurdle. What's next is choosing a diet. While you don't have to be an expert, taking a little extra time and care to select your personal weight-loss regime can balance the odds for success in your favor. You'll end up with the diet that works best because it's right for you.

Choosing a diet can be a little like buying a dress off the racks. High-protein or low-carbohydrate? Grapefruit or cottage cheese? Dr. Stillman, Dr. Atkins or Dr. Kempner? Calories or grams? Water, milk or wine? Vegetables? Better yet, no food at all? Sorting through them all is as confusing to most of us as confronting the new line of fall fashions. All you want, after a while, is a personal diet shopper, someone to say, "Here, Mrs. Yatzy, this diet's going to look absolutely great on you."

Experimenting is one way to go about it, but if you're serious about slimming, I honestly don't recommend the dabble technique. Some diets will be disastrous for you, and after coming to this conclusion five or six times, you won't want to try again. I remember one particular year when, faced with a scale that put me over the mark by 15 pounds, I ran through six different diets before

DESIRABLE WEIGHT CHART

	HEIGHT (without shoes)	SMALL FRAME	MEDIUM FRAME	LARGE FRAME
WOMEN	5 ft. 0 in.	92- 98	96-107	104-109
	5 ft. 1 in.	94-101	98-110	106-112
	5 ft. 2 in.	96-104	101-113	109-118
	5 ft. 3 in.	99-107	104-116	112-121
	5 ft. 4 in.	102-110	107-119	115-125
	5 ft. 5 in.	105-113	110-122	118-130
	5 ft. 6 in.	108-116	113-126	121-135
	5 ft. 7 in.	111-119	116-130	125-140
	5 ft. 8 in.	114-123	120-135	129-145
	5 ft. 9 in.	118-127	124-139	133-150
	5 ft. 10 in.	122-131	128-143	137-155
	5 ft. 11 in.	126-135	132-147	141-160
	6 ft. 0 in.	130-140	136-151	145-165
MEN	5 ft. 4 in.	115-123	121-133	129-132
	5 ft. 5 in.	118-126	124-136	132-137
	5 ft. 6 in.	121-129	127-139	135-142
	5 ft. 7 in.	124-133	130-143	138-148
	5 ft. 8 in.	128-137	134-147	142-152
	5 ft. 9 in.	132-141	138-152	147-155
	5 ft. 10 in.	136-145	142-156	151-160
	5 ft. 11 in.	140-150	146-160	155-165
	6 ft. 0 in.	144-154	150-165	159-170
	6 ft. 1 in.	148-158	154-170	164-175
	6 ft. 2 in.	152-162	158-175	168-180
	6 ft. 3 in.	156-167	162-180	173-185
	6 ft. 4 in.	160-171	167-185	178-190

concluding that fate had simply not meant for me to be thin. I dropped the whole idea for another helping of chocolate cake—and another two seasons.

There *are* shortcuts to success. Evaluating a diet in terms of your own individual needs before blindly jumping into it can pre-warn you of any number of reasons it might be unsuitable, and therefore unsuccessful. Why, for instance, stock your freezer with two weeks' of high-protein ammunition when you're the type who can't give up sweets? Sweets are prohibited on most high-protein diets and I guarantee you'll start craving them not two days into the diet. Or, if you are an exuberant, undisciplined gal, the life of every party, why harness yourself by counting calories? Too cautious for *your* personality. Knowing things like this beforehand helps.

Aside from willpower, there are four "diet success factors," which, if analyzed carefully, will guide you straight to the perfect diet. They are: *your food preferences, your personality traits, your life-style and the reasons you're overweight*. I'll go through them one by one. Regardless of how well you already know yourself, take this diet self-analysis test. It's a quickie—all you need is pencil, paper and the desire to be beautifully thin!

1. *Food preferences:* Strictly a matter of individual taste. The foods your man loves—meat, potatoes, bacon and eggs—may be ones you could easily live without, while he, on the other hand, might be delighted to forego your favorite vegetables, fruits and ice cream. It's all according to your personality. While some lucky few can lock up the sweets cupboard with nary a qualm, others need to have that sugar goodie treat every day. I'm a starch and sugar fiend myself, with a penchant for baked potatoes, chocolate ice cream, fresh bread and Mallomars—a throwback to childhood. Without them I feel utterly deprived. I've learned over the years that a diet which excludes these passion foods is a real struggle. The strange thing is, when I know they're allowed on my diet, I never go overboard. Childish, yes, but I guess it's all in feeling you can make the decision for yourself.

With pencil and paper, profile your own eating habits. First list those foods you eat regularly during the course of a week. Don't neglect ingredients like butter, cream, whipped cream, sugar and oils if you cook with them. Also inventory all snacks, treats and eat-out items like pizza, custard, tacos and quick burgers with French fries. In a diet, they can put you right over the top.

After you've completed the list, read through it, again with pencil in hand. Now cross out those foods you think you could give up. Don't be ultra-virtuous. If you really adore a particular food—chocolate sundaes, for example—don't eliminate it because you'd like to believe it's unimportant to you. Keep it on the list: there's a diet that makes allowances for ice cream lovers.

You're ready now to analyze your food preferences. Which foods seem prevalent? If sugars and starches, fruits and vegetables are can't-do-withouts, you're asking for trouble on a low-carbohydrate diet where those come under the "forbidden" or "limited" heading. Try one of the low-calorie diets instead, where breads and pasta—even strawberry shortcake—are permitted now and again. Your sweet tooth will be satisfied and so will your desire for a skinnier shape. For lovers of meats, fish, cream and oil, there's no diet more comfortable than a low-carbohydrate plan. Make the most of your natural inclinations by counting grams. It's quick, for the most part, and you'll hardly even notice you're dieting. Keep your food list by your side as you read through the diets section. Circle the diet or diets that conform to your own specific tastes.

2. *Personality traits:* There is no sense selecting a diet that goes against your grain. Matching diet to personality is another safeguard against backsliding. If, for instance, you're a fast-mover (I'm one) and like to see instant results for your efforts, dropping one or two pounds a week will frustrate the daylights out of you; you'd do better crashing for the first week, or following a super-low calorie diet for dramatic results. Check either (a) or (b) for each of the following questions, depending on which statement best describes you:

1. (a) I am a fairly patient person.
   (b) I like to see quick results when I do something.
2. (a) I think of myself as conservative.
   (b) I love drama and mystery in my life.
3. (a) I am a fastidious housekeeper.
   (b) I am not fussy about my home.
4. (a) I have been on a diet only once before.
   (b) I have dieted many times before.
5. (a) I am very good at budgeting.
   (b) I am an impulse shopper.
6. (a) I want to lose weight for a specific reason.
   (b) I just want to lose weight—period.
7. (a) I like keeping to a schedule.
   (b) I usually don't like schedules.
8. (a) I am pretty even-tempered.
   (b) I have a quick temper.
9. (a) I am an habitual list-maker.
   (b) I don't like to write anything down.
10. (a) I am basically a realist.
    (b) I am a romantic at heart.
11. (a) I want to lose 5–10 pounds.
    (b) I want to lose more than 10 pounds.
12. (a) I don't mind the idea of dieting.
    (b) I hate to diet.

Check through your answers. If they were mostly (a), a low-calorie diet would probably suit you best. Low-calorie diets, most of which are relatively slower-working than low-carbo plans, are a good match for your essentially calm nature. You won't have a problem sticking to the rules, nor being watchful about counting calories. One of the diets in the low-calorie section should suit you to a tee. If most of the answers you checked were (b), you'd undoubtedly do very, very well on one of the low-carbohydrate weight-loss plans. Not so strict as low-cal diets, low-carbo plans don't limit your intake of certain foods—so you, who don't like restraints, won't feel deprived. These diets work fast, another point in their favor. You'll actually be able to see a noticeable figure change within a week.

A word on crash diets and fasting. Who should go on these? Any healthy individual who wants to see an immediate, dramatic weight loss. Because your intake is so severely restricted, you will lose upwards of five pounds per week on most crash diets. They're super for getting you off to a good start if you have lots of excess flab to get rid of. Remember, though, just one week on a crash diet, and not more than a few days on a liquid fast! As with every diet, check with your doctor first.

3. *Your lifestyle:* Depending upon whether you spend your days at home or at a 9 to 5 office job, your diet requirements will vary. In choosing a diet, think about your regular habits. Are you at home during the day, and thus able to follow a strict eating plan? Perhaps you are a career person who needs more diet flexibility? Some people dine out regularly. If you do, you'll want to plan a diet that encompasses the menu of your favorite restaurant. A life-style that includes a great deal of entertaining makes still other demands—select a diet that's adaptable enough for you to join your guests at the table. Moreover, cooking for a husband and children means your diet will have to be worked around family meals, for convenience's sake as well as for the sake of the budget. You know your life-style better than anyone else. Be aware that your diet will be smooth sailing if it fits within your normal patterns. Again, make a list of these. Keep it handy as you search for your perfect diet.

4. *Reasons you're overweight:* This last one is the ringer. For most people with a weight problem, coming to terms with the cause or causes for overeating is as unpleasant as a trip to the dentist. Not only is it painful to admit such things as insecurity, anger or frustration, but the root causes may lie buried under years of rationalizing and excuse-making. It will probably take some hard thinking to pinpoint them at all. Still, I believe knowing why you eat too much will help make you stop doing it. Understanding is one of the first keys to slimming success. Consider the real reasons you overeat—thinking about it is bound to be uncomfortable at times, but remember, so is being heavy.

People overeat for different reasons, and practically

none of them have to do with hunger. In fact, psychologists tell us that the majority of obese people don't even know when they are hungry. The act of putting food in the mouth has other symbolic value far removed from either taste or appetite. For most overweights, the pattern begins at a very young age as part of the child's learning process—gone slightly haywire.

Remember hearing, "That's Mama's good little darling!" as a sweet candy was popped into your adorable little mouth? You'd just gotten an "A" on a spelling test or had finally been talked out of beating up little brother for smashing your favorite toy. That lollipop, or whatever it was, came as a reward for "acceptable behavior," and you, quite logically (children are eminently logical), drew the conclusion: good = reward = food, a formula that's stuck until this day. So now when you do something "good" (as an adult it's likely to be a success on the job, getting through a difficult social situation or keeping the family fed, clothed and happy), you go back to that same reward system. You treat yourself to another helping of your favorite food. If you're good again, yet another helping.

By the same token, many parents withdraw special treats as punishment when a child has misbehaved. Instead of stopping to discover why a child may have acted the way he or she did, a harried parent may deliver this (familiar?) edict: "O.K. This time no dessert tonight." All grown up, that same child may engage in chronic rebellion against this punishment, unconsciously reasoning: "Hey, there's nobody to stop me now. I can eat whatever I want to!"

Some parents are born worriers, overprotective of little ones for what they consider to be good cause. One of my cousins was a casualty of such a sheltered upbringing. As a child, Michael was prevented from doing a lot of things other kids were allowed to do. He couldn't go outside when it was raining or snowing (he'd catch pneumonia); nor could he play in the sun without a shirt (he'd burn); playing on the playground monkey bars was strictly forbidden (he'd fall to his death); and he couldn't get closer than ten feet to a dog (rabies, you know). What Michael could do, in case you're wondering, was eat. The more, the better. Why? Because layers of fat, according to my aunt, were protection against disease. All plump and rosy-cheeked, Michael was safe from those omnipresent "germs." A successful lawyer today, with a lovely wife and two children, my cousin Michael, until three years ago, was obese. You see, all his life he'd had this constant fear of getting terribly sick if he didn't eat a lot . . . see what I mean? Those elementary lessons are unlearned with difficulty and pain. In Michael's case, it took some months with a professional therapist.

There's no doubt that many children associate food with love and security. It's a connection learned at the mother's breast where, warm and safe, the infant's first desires are instantly gratified. The baby cries and it is fed. Immediate wants are taken care of and all is well. All is secure. In adulthood, one's wants and needs are more complex, harder to satisfy. Most of the time, we must work out solutions for ourselves and with no more mother there to anticipate our every need, we revert to the memory of what once satisfied us completely: food. Eating creates the illusion of total security.

And since food is love, maternal love specifically, overeating is what we do when there are kinks in our own love lives. Problems within a relationship, lack of a current romantic interest, separation and divorce—all these are "cured" with food. In fact, chronic fatties use food as an antidote to loneliness in general—a remedy which, sadly, never works, since the heavier they get, the more reluctant they are to make contact with people and the lonelier they become. Constant eating anesthetizes the loneliness and the need for love, at least for a little while.

Unusually obese individuals may go into hiding behind a "wall of flesh," usually because they feel bad about themselves and don't want anyone to come too close. Beneath an outward façade of joviality, many heavy people are actually alone and quite frightened. Or they may feel that being physically bigger makes them more important; in reality, they see themselves as small and insignificant. In such extreme cases, professional counseling may be useful in combatting the problem.

We are all different. We may eat because we're hungry. We *over*eat because we're anxious, afraid, sad, upset, bored, frustrated, guilty, lonely, depressed, angry—each of us for our own private reasons. It takes a lot of undoing to change patterns of a lifetime. They're ingrained at a deep, deep level of awareness so that we hardly even know they're operating. Attempting to alter these patterns is well worth the effort. Before you choose your diet plan, give these ideas, strange though they may seem to you, some serious thought. No matter the diet, it will help you to understand why you've needed to overeat in the past.

By now, you should be prepared to select your diet plan. To ensure that you'll be marvelously successful and, within a few short weeks, as sleek and attractive as you want to be, I've assembled a few hints, tips and diet tricks from notebooks I've filled over the years. Whether you're following a low-carbo, low-cal or crash plan, they apply to you.

Do not attempt to diet if:
- You are unduly emotionally upset.
- You are going through a change in your life—moving, switching jobs, marriage, divorce, visit from out-of-town guests or relatives.
- You are on a vacation.
- The holidays are just around the corner.
- You are quitting smoking.
- You are ill.

Each of these conditions is unusually demanding in its own way. Thus preoccupied, you'll have little time and less energy for the special strains of dieting. Wait for calmer times, when your chances of success are greatest by far. If you've cleared these conditions, however, you can start your diet tomorrow. And you should. I find that as the gap between intention and action widens, I'm likely to be distracted by other "more important" projects.

You may want to develop your own dieting scheme,

a set of workable guidelines to guarantee that your diet is a smashing success. The Seven Diet Rules which follow are my own. I follow them whenever I need to lose weight, whichever diet I decide on. Perhaps you will want to use them as a point of departure for creating your own diet rules.

CORINNE'S SEVEN DIET RULES

1. *Decide how many pounds you want to lose.* Pick an exact number. Write it down on a piece of paper and pin the paper up somewhere in full view. The refrigerator door is the best spot in the house. Or tack that magic number up in more than one place if you need special reminding.

2. *Choose a diet that's suitable for you.* If you've read everything that's gone before this, finding your super diet will be a snap. Once you've found it, don't switch until you've given it two weeks' fair chance. But if, after that time, you've concluded it's unworkable, simply choose another diet and go with *it*. Give your diet every chance to succeed with a positive I-can-do-it attitude.

3. *Reward yourself each week for weight loss.* I believe in rewards. If there's anyone who needs them, it's the nibbler deprived of an eating habit. At the end of each week, go out and buy yourself a little something for being so good. It needn't be anything extravagant— a small houseplant, a pretty bracelet, a good book or a new lipstick will make you feel extra-special.

4. *Change your self-image right now.* Slim and shapely, that's what you are! You're not a fattie anymore, but if you continue to see yourself that way, you'll be working against your diet. Develop an image of yourself that's positively positive. Reinforce your slender image by packing away part of your oversized wardrobe. Stick with just a few attractive fashions, clothes you like. As pounds start to melt away, take in your clothing so it fits. For incentive, purchase a dress in the size you want to be and keep trying it on until it

zips without tugging. Keep tabs on your progress with a daily mirror check—watch those bulges disappear.

5. *Stick to your diet, no matter what.* It takes will-power and resolution, often in the face of overwhelming temptation. Be aware of your own weaknesses, whether those moments comes at a friend's home for dinner, late at night in front of the TV or midmorning when you're alone at home. Catch yourself before you can say "just this once." At times when you feel temptation nagging at your morale, begin some other activity to take your mind off food. Pick up your needlepoint or patchwork, furiously clean the bathroom, even leave the house if you must. The urge will pass, and soon, so will the frequency of your cravings. At the point of giving in, I talk to myself aloud: "You don't really want that pie, do you? No, of course not. You're doing great. Look at how much weight you've lost already! You want to lose some more, don't you? You're thin!" I've become expert in the art of self-persuasiveness, though I'm not quite sure what the neighbors think.

6. *Reward yourself for reaching your diet goal.* Having reached your desirable weight, go out and celebrate with a well-earned gift for yourself. Splurge with something you've always wanted—after all, you *do* deserve it. Then, get right back on your diet and lose two more pounds. Consider these as diet insurance. This way, if you gain an extra pound, you won't feel terrible about it.

7. *Develop a maintenance diet to stay on forever.* Yes, you're fat prone and, unfortunately, you probably will be all your life. Eating whatever you want to just because you've lost weight will only send the scales rocketing back up again. Instead, work out a sensible maintenance plan, one you can stay on for the rest of your life. Rules can be relaxed a bit now, but not eliminated. Be sure your eating plan works in terms of your life-style and particular needs.

Just a few more footnotes . . . every dieter should anticipate pitfalls and setbacks along the way. They happen to the best of us and shouldn't be any cause to feel you've failed. Some common ones are:

The two-week plateau: for most dieters, relatively

fewer pounds are lost during the third week of a diet, which many regard as personal failure. Not true. Much of the weight lost during the first and second week is water weight. During the third week, what you're losing is more actual fat, which is slower to disappear. Don't quit! Rather, cut eating down an extra bit to give yourself a push off the plateau.

Lack of encouragement from others: Yes, it's true. Even very good friends may not want to see you get thin. Often, they are overweights who have never managed a successful diet themselves. Sometimes it's because they don't want a good friend to change. Avoid those people who are likely to chip away at your determination.

Nervousness and irritability: Common with dieters, who are trading comfortable old habits for unfamiliar new ones. To alleviate a case of diet nerves, try this calmer-downer: hie yourself to the quietest spot in the house, preferably a darkened bedroom, which is ideal. Undress or change into some loose-fitting clothing and lie down on the bed. Rest on your back, with arms at your sides, palms face up. Close your eyes. Begin to relax by taking very deep breaths: inhale through your nostrils, gathering in lots of air, so that chest, diaphragm and belly swell to fullness. Hold the breath for a count of five. Now exhale, very slowly, allowing every last bit of air to escape through your mouth. Continue deep breathing in this manner, at the same time clearing your mind of all thoughts. Just concentrate on relaxing your whole body. I personally guarantee this simple exercise as one of the world's best muscle and mind soothers.

Fears: Even as you diet, you may be beset by fears of one sort or another. Fear of your body changing, fear of what friends and relatives will say about the "new" you, fear of dieting success, fear of being attractive and sexually desirable . . . not only are these normal, they're common. Don't let them dampen your spirits, simply push them out of your mind. In truth, losing weight will make you more content with yourself than you've ever been.

Breaking your diet: You will break your diet. The

odds are in favor of an occasional lapse here and there. Don't feel too guilty, but do get right back on your program. The longer you procrastinate, the more difficulty you'll have resuming.

To coin a phrase, on to the meat of the book—the actual diets themselves. Do read through them carefully, with your diet profile in hand. I'm absolutely certain you will find the one diet to slim you, trim you and really make that big, beautiful change you're looking for. Good luck!

THE DIETS

These diets work—that's why I've chosen them. Every one is a proven pound-peeler—a diet classic for an overweight crisis. Even if you've never been able to lose weight before, if you're a self-confessed flop at the diet game, there is at least one regime in this roundup that will allow you to take off as few or as many pounds as you wish. I promise. The diets are here. All you have to provide is the obstinate determination to be thin.

Choose one that's lightning-fast or go with a diet that shows more leisurely results. The proper pace is one you can live with most comfortably. Most diets included in this section are short-term, designed to remove excess weight within weeks. As I've said before, there's something here for everybody. Low-calorie, low-carbohydrate, crash diets, even group weight loss programs that match up perfectly with your taste buds and temperament.

Take a look at each of these classics before deciding which one you're going to follow. Armed with your diet profile, skim through them quickly to see which appeal to you at first glance. Don't ponder too much the first time around; you'll respond with an "Aha, I like that one," to plans which are compatible. Circle the diets you think you'd do well with. When you've read through the entire section, go back and look over the diets you've circled, this time more carefully. Weigh the plus and minus points of each in terms of *you*. I'll caution again: if, for example, you aren't a big morning eater, don't pick a diet that features hearty breakfasts. If you're a nibbler, go with one of the plans that lets you eat more than three times a day. If you're a sweets lover, reject any diet that prohibits sweets altogether. The ultimate success of your diet is directly related to how much sense it makes for you. When you're ready to, make your final choice. Pick the diet that's going to allow you to lose all that built-up fat once and forever.

I prefer to copy my diet onto a piece of paper where it's handy for reference, and perhaps you might find this useful. In fact, I usually make two copies, one for my refrigerator door and one for my pocketbook. This way I know what to buy when I go grocery shopping and what I can eat when dining out. On most diets, you'll be counting either calories or grams. Invest in a small spiral notebook to record your diet progress (you can also copy your diet into it). Note your weight goal, daily calorie or gram limits and, most importantly, every single gram or calorie—whichever you're watching—that passes your lips. Remember, you must write down everything you eat, even such forgettables as the half-pat of butter on your bread or that mint candy you took from a friend. In the diet game, all these little pieces add up. At the end of each day, total your intake. If you're over the mark, resolve to do better tomorrow. Chart your progressive weight loss, too. Seeing the numbers decrease from week to week is marvelous incentive.

Again, I urge you to see your doctor for a complete physical before you begin your diet. It goes without saying that you should be in good health before undertaking a weight loss. Any diet is change—and any change is somewhat stressful for the body. Furthermore, your doctor will be able to detect problems that may be contributing to a weight problem, if they exist. *Tell* your doctor you're about to diet—and do describe the plan you've chosen.

Finally, five additional hints that apply to every dieter. Follow them, and the road to success will be happy and healthful.

- Take a multivitamin every day.
- Get adequate sleep.
- Drink plenty of water.
- Limit your intake of salt.
- Avoid overly strenuous exercise.*

* Each of you knows your own limits. Don't overdo it!

You're on your way to a slim new figure. As exasperating as dieting is for you, resolve to stick with it. If you go off your diet, go right back on it again. Take it from one who's been on both sides of the fat fence—thin is definitely better.

THE LOW-CALORIE DIETS

Anyone who has ever tried to reduce knows what a low-calorie diet is. More than likely, you've done your own fair share of calorie counting at some point or another—especially if you put on and take off pounds like a yo-yo. "195 calories for the half-can of tuna, 100 for the dollop of mayo, 56 for the slice of whole wheat bread . . ." Though not the world's most stimulating pastime, counting calories *is,* nonetheless, reliable. You will drop pounds, lose inches and banish unwanted fat if you cut your daily intake of calories. How much depends on the extent to which you can stand depriving your stomach.

Calories, as I've said, are a way of measuring the energy-producing value in food. Foods that are high in calories produce considerable energy; low-calorie foods produce less. Most of us overweights put on pounds because we don't use up all the energy produced by the calories we consume. That excess energy is stored in our bodies—chiefly as fat—and up goes the scale. To lose weight, we have to cut down on calories, thereby forcing our bodies to utilize body fat for energy.

To lose one pound of body weight, you must slice 3500 calories from your caloric intake. If you've got lots to lose, doctors and nutrition experts recommend a weekly weight loss of not more than two pounds, for safety's sake, although quicker-working plans and crashes are fine as a first-week morale booster for the novice dieter. Check with your own physician to be sure. In terms of calories, two pounds per week equals a daily cutback of 1000 calories. Thus, if your own daily requirement is 2000 calories, for example, limiting your intake to 1000 calories per day will show you two pounds thinner in just seven days.

Of course, you can work out your own personal low-calorie diet, including only those food favorites you want to eat. Simply set a calorie ceiling for yourself. Base it on the number of pounds you want to lose per week, and don't go over this magic number. The method works, yes, but I consider it a last resort. If you've exhausted every other diet, and none of them work, then by all means go ahead with your own plan. I know some successful slimmers who've done it with some pretty strange and wacky food combinations.

For most of us, however, the low-calorie diet classics are your best bet. They've worked for millions of dieters over the years, and they'll work for you. You can—you will—lose every last unwanted pound by paying close mind to the Grapefruit Diet's sunshine rules, the Rice Diet's oriental proscriptions or the pounds-off eccentricities of the famous American Hot Dog Diet, to name just a few. Your beautiful figure is just a calorie count away . . .

The Grapefruit Diet

The grapefruit diet dates back—at the very least—to 1941, when it appeared within the elegant pages of *Harper's Bazaar* as the Nine Day Wonder Diet, a weight loss plan for fashion-conscious women who needed to whisk pounds away quickly. Since that time, many reducing plans have been billed as grapefruit diets; *Bazaar* itself reprinted their 1941 diet in 1971 as the Diet for the Midi. The midi's had its ups and downs, but the diet lives on, still working its slimming miracles. This version, as far as I can tell, is the original grapefruit diet, *grand-mère* of them all.

You can expect to lose nine pounds on the plan, a pound a day for the nine days the diet lasts. The delectable mainstays of this diet are grapefruit, meat, eggs and, oddly enough, tomatoes. However, you are not limited to these foods. This is a balanced eating program which includes vegetables, fruit, salad and even an occasional sandwich! *Bazaar* author Elinor Guthrie Neff offered two pieces of advice for the first grapefruit dieters: *don't* partake of any liquor (alcohol will slow weight loss considerably) and *do* eat heartily; relishing your food is one of the least-publicized secrets of successful dieting.

THE GRAPEFRUIT DIET MENUS

As you read through the following menus, don't be intimidated by the very exact portions called for in some instances. Should you go over the amount specified—if, for example, you have four and a half ounces of steak instead of four—the world won't fall apart. And your diet will still work. Though *Bazaar* did not give specific portions, I have, since this is not a low-carbo diet and calories *do* count.

Breakfast: Wake up each morning to the same sunshine breakfast: one whole medium-sized grapefruit and a piping hot cup of black coffee or tea.

Lunch: You get a choice here, but do follow these menu guidelines to a tee:

   3 lunches: 2 large eggs; 3 saltines
   2 lunches: 2 oz. chicken, 1 oz. ham or 1 oz. cheese sandwich on rye bread
   3 lunches: 4 oz. meat, minute steak, cubed steak or 2 small lamb chops; 1 cup stewed tomatoes
   1 lunch: French toast

On one lucky afternoon, you may round your luncheon meal out with the appetizer of your choice, any additional vegetable and a half-serving of your favorite dessert. For a second midday dessert, you may have one medium-sized apple.

Dinner: Dinner offers variety, too. Enjoy these tempting low-calorie main meals:

   3 dinners: 5 oz. sirloin or tenderloin steak; endive and tomato salad; 1 cup wax or string beans
   2 dinners: two 4½ oz. lamb chops; lettuce and cucumber salad; 1 sliced tomato
   1 dinner: 5 oz. ground round; mixed green salad; 1 cup spinach or 8 asparagus spears

1 dinner: 6 oz. broiled halibut; 1 cup raw, shredded cabbage; 1 cup cauliflower; 1 cup carrots

1 dinner: 2 eggs; 1 cup stewed tomatoes; 1 cup brussels sprouts

For dessert each evening, serve yourself a good-sized half grapefruit. Feel free to mix and match salads and vegetables as you please, but keep to the rules about main dishes.

Not permitted: Butter, mayonnaise, catsup, steak sauce or other common caloric condiments.

Permitted: Unlimited quantities of water, calorie-free soft drinks, bouillon, black coffee or tea with lemon.

Cooking tips: Though *Bazaar* didn't specify how to cook your eggs, I suggest using a non-stick pan (no fat, please) for scrambled eggs or omelette; or prepare by poaching, baking or soft-cooking. Eggs take on wonderfully shaded flavor if you add a dash of your favorite herb to them before cooking—oregano adds zest, chives add piquancy, pepper adds bite.

Be experimental with herbs in preparing vegetables, too. Just the tiniest amounts add a festive touch to these side-dishes. Tomatoes, as anyone who's ever cooked Italian-style knows, are blessed by the addition of oregano, basil or thyme; cucumbers adore dill; and brussels sprouts and salads are infinitely more interesting with a sprinkle of caraway seeds. Improvise with selections from your own spice shelf.

Make your own tasty salad dressing—you'll love it even after these nine diet days are over—by combining vinegar or lemon juice with powdered mustard, seasoned salt and fresh-ground pepper to taste. Shake well, then sprinkle over crisp, cool salad greens.

Broil your meat and fish; before cooking, trim all visible fat from steaks and lamb chops. If you're eating in a restaurant, ask the waiter to remove all fat before serving you.

A final note on grapefruits: for variety, try broiling a half-grapefruit. Just a few minutes under the fire transforms this health fruit into a hot, tangy gourmet treat.

The Nibbling Diet

McCall's called it the Snack Diet and reported its success in 1963 and again in 1970. In 1964, *Vogue* dubbed it the Nibbling Diet—"one of the seven most-talked-about diets of the moment." And people are still talking.

On the Nibbling Diet, you eat six meals a day—yes, six: It's a low-calorie plan developed by doctors, who rely on it widely themselves when they want to shed excess poundage. According to its fans, it is the only low-calorie plan that truly satisfies hunger.

If you're wondering how anyone can possibly reduce when they're constantly eating, be assured that there's logic behind the method: by consuming six small meals a day, you force your body to utilize more stored-up fat than it does when you consume the *same* number of calories in three large meals. That's the theory, and although there's no absolute evidence to back it up, the Nibbling Diet has been effective in numerous controlled medical experiments. The best-known of these were by Dr. Edgar S. Gordon of the University of Wisconsin Medical Center. While nibbling six meals—and 1320 calories—a day, 80 of Dr. Gordon's overweight patients lost an average of 10 to 14 pounds a month!

THE NIBBLING DIET MENUS

The Nibbling Diet is not for everyone. To follow it, your schedule must allow you to eat at these six intervals: morning, mid-morning, noon, mid-afternoon, early evening and late evening. If you cannot eat at these times—for example, if your job doesn't permit a mid-morning or mid-afternoon break—this *isn't* the diet for you.

All your meals—all six of them—must be about the same size. All must include foods taken from the following group:

lean meat, poultry, fish, seafood; skim-milk cottage cheese; plain yogurt; eggs; cheese; fresh fruit; green and other non-starchy vegetables; bread; polyunsaturated fats

(Note that you may not have more than half a slice of bread daily; and not more than a tablespoon daily of polyunsaturated fats.)

The Nibbling Diet is a low-calorie plan whose success depends on limiting the number of calories you take in each day. On this diet, it is necessary to count calories very carefully, and for this, as I've suggested before, it might be helpful to record everything you eat in a small spiral notebook.

The number of calories you consume each day will determine the rapidity of your weight loss. If you're impatient, you might limit yourself to 1000 calories a day; if you are comfortable with a slower diet pace, allow yourself up to, but not more than, 1300 calories. But remember, no matter what limitations you set for yourself, eat only the permitted foods and keep your six meals just about equal in size.

Take a good look at the sample menu plan below. It's based on intaking less than 1100 clories, spread evenly over six nibbling meals. Use it as an aid in developing your own diet meals.

Morning
½ medium banana
1 soft-cooked egg
½ slice white toast

Mid-morning
1 oz. Swiss cheese
1 whole tomato

Noon
4 oz. broiled chicken
1 cup green beans

Mid-afternoon
½ cup plain yogurt
1 cup fresh strawberries

Evening
4 oz. broiled ground round

1 cup cauliflower
½ cucumber, sliced

Mid-evening
1 oz. American cheese
¼ medium cantaloupe

Nibbling at this rate, you should take off 10 pounds in less than three weeks, without needless suffering and hunger.

Not permitted: Anything *not* included on the Nibbling Diet foods list!

Permitted: Unlimited quantities of water, calorie-free soft drinks, bouillon, black coffee, tea with lemon.

Cooking tips: Try to vary your nibble-meals. There are an enormous number of interesting foods permitted within the basic outline of this diet, so be adventurous! Try fish and seafood you've never had before—many people, for example, consider raw cherrystone clams on the half-shell a real delicacy. There are unusual vegetables available on your greengrocer's shelf, too: kale, beet greens, bean sprouts, arrugula (an aromatic salad green which tastes like it has salad dressing *in* it) and okra are a delicious departure from more common fare. Don't get into a rut by preparing the same foods all the time. You'll be bored in no time at all—and that spells danger to any dieter.

Diet hints: Though meals are mini-sized, don't be mini-minded about eating them. Treat each of your six meals as if it were a full-course dinner. Set an attractive place setting every time you eat, complete with mat, silver, napkin, and water glass. Serving each food on a different dish makes the meal seem even more lavish, and I promise you it will last longer. Rest your fork on your plate while you're chewing, and don't pick it up again until you are actually ready for the next bite. Not only will this make the food last longer, but it'll also force you into really tasting what you're eating. In short, don't gobble your food down—even if the diet is designed for nibblers.

The Rice Diet

People have been writing about rice diets for over 25 years, and they all invariably begin with, "Have you ever seen an overweight Oriental?" Well, frankly, yes! I used to take cooking classes from a Chinese gentleman who looked as if he was making nightly raids on the refrigerator for third and fourth helpings of egg roll and chop suey. But I'll grant that plump Orientals are a rarity because Asian cooking is skinny cooking. And not only are the foods filling, they also taste good.

The most famous rice diet in this country was developed in the 1940s by Dr. Walter Kempner of Duke University. It was originally designed for patients with heart and kidney disorders, but the diet proved so effective that it was soon adopted by thousands of overweights from coast to coast. Since the plan's inception a quarter century ago, it has been used at the Duke Clinic to help reduce over 6000 overweight men and women.

Variations of the Kempner abound, but the one I like best appeared in *Coronet* in January 1960. Enticingly, it was titled the No-Hunger Rice Diet. The plan, adapted to American tastes, combines Chinese and American-style cooking and offers an infinite variety of exotic foods and flavors. If you love to eat, you'll love this diet.

THE RICE DIET MENUS

Let me begin by saying that you can expect to lose at least 10 pounds in 12 days on this version of the rice diet. You'll lose even more by skimping at dinner, where lean meat and poultry may be added to the regular menu.

Take a trip to your local market to stock up on the exotic seasonings that lend unique taste to Oriental cookery: ginger, anise, tumeric, coriander and clove (sometimes packaged together as "five spice powder") are basics. Invest in some authentic soy sauce (most flavorful is the Japanese *Shoyu* sauce, which you can eas-

ily find in most supermarkets) or canned bamboo
shoots, bean sprouts, meatless chow mein and Chinese
vegetables, which come either canned or frozen-style.
And don't forget the rice, either natural brown or long-
grain white. Forget precooked rice, which has less tex-
ture and, in most cases, more calories.

Prepare for your 10-day diet by cooking large quantities of rice in advance. Two and a half cups of raw rice
makes seven and a half cups of cooked rice, a three-day
supply. Before cooking, wash the rice thoroughly in a
sieve held under cold running water and rinse until the
water runs clear. Let the rice cook (without salt!), then
refrigerate in a plastic container with a tight lid.

Breakfast: Breakfast every day is a half-cup of rice
with a full cup of fresh fruit: strawberries, blueberries,
raspberries, diced cantaloupe, banana or peach slices,
orange or grapefruit sections. Sprinkle with cinnamon
for extra flavor.

Lunch: A whole cup of rice, heated in a double
boiler or by steaming, with one full cup of Chinese
mixed vegetables or meatless chow mein. Season before
heating with a teaspoon or two of soy sauce and a pinch
of spice. You may, if you like, substitute any low-
calorie vegetable for the Chinese-style greens. Mushrooms, broccoli, spinach and stewed tomatoes are all
tempting complements to your daily rice bowl. Season
vegetables with herbs and a tiny dab of butter.

Dinner: A repeat of lunch: rice and Chinese-style or
plain vegetables, except that for your evening meal you
may add three ounces of any lean broiled meat (make
sure to trim off all visible fat) or four ounces of cooked
chicken (with skin removed) or lobster. If you add
meat, slice it razor-fine. Dice or chunk-cut chicken.
Mix all ingredients together in a double boiler and season to taste before heating.

On this super low-calorie diet, your intake is limited
to fewer than 950 calories per day and, if you're like
most people who try it, you'll find there's more here to
eat than you'll be able to finish. Refrigerate leftovers—
who knows, you may be hungry after an hour or so!

Cooking tips: Vegetables cooked by steaming retain both flavor and crunchiness, also more of their vitamins. If you don't own a steamer, set vegetables in an ordinary strainer over a pot of boiling water. Cover and let steam for a few minutes.

Diet hints: Eat with chopsticks, like the Chinese do. Getting the knack of it isn't really difficult, all it requires is a bit of patience. By taking smaller mouthfuls, which chopsticks force you to do, meals will last longer, food will seem much tastier and your scale will take a giant plunge downward.

As a special treat, eat one diet rice meal out at a Chinese restaurant. Order a dish of exotic vegetables not available on your supermarket shelf, or try special beef, chicken and lobster dishes prepared in the chef's unique style. And do sip that delicious Chinese tea. You can have cup after cup after cup without worrying a bit about your waistline!

The Career Girl's Diet

Working women have a notoriously bad time dieting. What with mid-morning and afternoon coffee breaks, noon-time lunches at the local coffee shop, plus the tendency of the desk-bound to munch on candy bars, pretzels and potato chips (a diversion that seems to make the time to go faster), losing weight is like battling a tidal wave. This diet, devised by a group of New York career women to take care of their collective fanny spread, will let you lose weight on the job. Many of my friends have had fantastic success with it, and I can report that I've lost many pounds following it, too.

This low-calorie plan limits you to less than 1200 calories per day, so that you should be able to see a loss of at least two pounds by the end of each week. Meals are simple and easy to fix, an important consideration for career people. The danger to working gals, of course, is the weekend. That burst of freedom you feel at 5 p.m. on Friday afternoons should *not* be celebrated with food. Treat yourself to an early movie with a friend or get home and into a nice, warm bath to make you feel good.

THE CAREER GIRL'S DIET MENUS

In this diet, there are three basic daily menus which you should eat on a rotating basis. You may, of course, mix and match breakfasts, lunches and dinners to suit your own tastes. The lunches include foods found on the menus of most coffee shops and restaurants.

MENU #1

Breakfast: 1 cup orange or unsweetened grapefruit juice; 1 egg (prepared without butter); 1 slice dry toast; black coffee or tea.

Lunch: Open-face turkey, chicken or roast-beef sandwich; lettuce and tomato salad; black coffee or tea.

Dinner: Broiled or baked fish; 2 vegetables from the list below; ½ cup rice; black coffee or tea.

MENU #2

Breakfast: 1 medium apple; ¾ cup cottage or pot cheese; 1 slice dry toast; black coffee or tea.

Lunch: Hamburger on a bun; 1 medium tomato; cole slaw; black coffee or tea.

Dinner: Broiled or boiled chicken; 2 vegetables from the list below; tossed green salad (low-calorie dressing); black coffee or tea.

MENU #3

Breakfast: ½ grapefruit; high-protein (unsweetened) dry cereal with skim milk; black coffee or tea.

Lunch: Fresh fruit salad or tuna fish platter; 1 slice dry toast; black coffee or tea.

Dinner: Up to 4 ounces steak, lamb chops, or veal; 2 vegetables from the list below; 1 small potato, boiled or baked; black coffee or tea.

For each dinner meal, choose *two* vegetables from among these: spinach, broccoli, carrots, beets, summer squash, zucchini, bean sprouts, cauliflower, tomatoes, collards, kale, okra, cabbage or mustard greens.

You may enjoy these snacks each day, also, one in the morning, and the second in the afternoon:

Mid-morning snack: 2 slices melba toast or 1 cup plain yogurt; black coffee or tea.

Mid-afternoon snack: 1 piece fresh fruit: apple, peach, pear, orange, tangerine, nectarine or plum.

Not permitted: Any food not included in the three basic menu plans.

Permitted: Unlimited quantities of water, calorie-free soft drinks, bouillon, black coffee, tea with lemon. Also, one teaspoon of butter, margarine or mayonnaise daily.

Cooking tips: The longer you cook beef, fish and poultry, the easier they are to digest—and the fewer calories they contain. Cook to medium or well-done.

Diet hints: For the duration of your diet, plan to have lunch with a friend who is also dieting. You can boost one another's morale while sticking to your regimes. If you go out to eat with other friends, don't mention that you're trying to lose weight. Your diet, and every diet story anyone can remember, will be the subject of conversation for the entire meal. This plan's "permitted" foods won't give you away, either—meals are so "normal" that no one will detect you're doing anything different.

Other lunching-out hints: tell your waiter not to bring the bread and butter. There's no use setting temptation right before your nose. Order salad without the house dressing every restaurant seems to be famous for. A squeeze of lemon or a little mustard mixed with vinegar will add plenty of tang to your bowl of leafy greens and keep you under your calorie limit at the same time.

The Hot Dog Diet

If your biggest problem on a diet—any diet, whether low-cal, low-carb or crash—is bread, or rather giving up bread, take a crack at my version of the *Look* (August 1963) Hot Dog Diet. For folks whose love of life is the staff of life, this is one of the great answers to near-painless reducing. And I mean that (excuse the pun) frankly.

As you might have guessed, the mainstays of this

plan are hot dogs and bread, but it's important that you pinpoint exactly the kind and size of both to stay within the diet. You must eat only pure-beef franks (kosher or non-kosher, take your pick), and you must not eat more than six ounces of dogs per day. If this sounds stunningly complicated, it isn't. Pure-beef franks are commonly sold in a one-pound package, containing eight or 10 franks. In the former instance, the weight per frank is two ounces; in the latter, 1.6 ounces. Multiply these figures by three—the number of hot dogs you're going to eat per day—and you'll find that you don't go over the number of ounces allowed.

Now for the hot dog rolls—which you aren't allowed to eat. They're far too calorie-expensive for this diet. Instead, wrap your frank in a slice of packaged white bread or, if you prefer, whole wheat bread. Larger sized bread slices, of course, will cost you more calories, sandwich-sized slices, fewer. The choice is yours, only be sure your total intake doesn't exceed 1000 calories per day.

THE HOT DOG DIET MENUS

Hot Dog Diet meals are no one's idea of gourmet eating. But they are fun if you think of your diet as an extended picnic, and they require little fuss or time in the kitchen. Should you tire of the menus given here, don't be afraid to invent your own. Again, don't go over the 1000 calories you're allowed each day.

Breakfast: Begin each day with a half-cup of skimmed milk, one soft-cooked egg or one ounce of cheese, and one low-calorie fruit: a peach or quarter of cantaloupe in summer, a tangerine or half-grapefruit in winter.

Lunch: This meal marks the start of your picnic. Choose from any of the combinations below; if you close your eyes, it's almost the Fourth of July!

1 frank, wrapped in bread;
½ cup sauerkraut; 2 large black olives

1 frank, wrapped in bread;
1 cup pickled green beans; 1 big dill pickle

1 frank, wrapped in bread;
1 whole tomato; 3 large green olives

1 frank, wrapped in bread;
1 cup cabbage slaw*; 1 sweet pickle stick

You must cook franks by boiling, broiling or grilling—frying is absolutely forbidden. To your hot dog, add any of the traditional (but low-calorie) trimmings: mustard, chopped onions, sauerkraut, hot peppers, etc.

Dinner: Dinner is two franks, again cooked by boiling, broiling or grilling; a small green salad; and one fruit, chosen from the breakfast list. You may have either two slices of bread with your franks, or alternatively, one slice of bread and a small helping of modified German potato salad.

Make the potato salad this way: boil one small potato in water to which you've added vinegar; drain; cut into very thin slices; sprinkle with chopped scallions, pepper, and a teaspoon of imitation bacon bits; serve warm.

Since your daily intake is limited to 900–1000 calories on the Hot Dog Diet, you can expect to lose five to eight pounds if you stay on it for a week to 10 days!

Cooking tips: I'd like to emphasize once more the importance of buying pure-beef franks, which have more protein value than other types of hot dogs. Even if beef franks are more expensive, which they usually are, the value is worth the few additional pennies.

Diet hints: The Hot Dog Diet, like the Nibble Diet, tempts one to forego eating at the table (I know I'm most used to nibbling franks standing up at baseball games or at picnics). Have your meal at the table, as you would if you weren't dieting. Eating on the run will only leave you with an unsatisfied feeling that will send you running to the 'fridge soon after you've finished your meal.

* Cooking note about cabbage slaw: fix it with vinegar, not mayonnaise. It's tangy that way and super low-calorie.

A general hint for dieters is appropriate here. Don't weigh yourself every day. Once or twice a week is plenty. Seeing no results or slow results is devastating for the dieter who's been good as gold and minded all the rules. It's a fact that none of us lose weight at a consistent rate; rather, your scale may show a pound lost for three days straight, then no change at all the next three days. Body chemistry sets the pace, and the body has its own reasons for a sporadic rate of loss. So, remember, once or twice a week on the scale and no more. You're sure to notice dramatic changes that way.

The Vegetable and Fruit Diet

Plato and Woody Allen; Gandhi and Robert Cummings; George Bernard Shaw and Dyan Cannon; Nehru and Efrem Zimbalist Jr. What do these uncommon people have in common? They are (or were) slender without effort. They are (or were) among the millions of people who practice day-in, day-out vegetarianism.

Of course, you don't have to be a full-fledged vegetarian to maintain a slim figure—there are other diets that will keep pounds off, too, and many of these include meat. But among diets, the Vegetable and Fruit Diet is one of the fastest routes to reducing, and should you get hooked on this pattern of eating, it's unlikely that you will ever be overweight again.

How much can you lose on the VFD? If you follow the plan faithfully for 14 days, you can expect to be trimmer by 10 to 14 pounds. If it turns out you want to continue vegetarianism, consult your doctor about balancing your diet to include sufficient amounts of protein.

THE VEGETABLE AND FRUIT DIET MENUS

Vegetables and fruits are the basics of this diet, but they are by no means the only foods you may eat. Each day you are allowed as well:

2 oz. any kind of cheese, cheese spread, or cheese food

1 cup soup: vegetable, onion, tomato, or mushroom (uncreamed)

1 slice bread and 4 saltines

5 tbsp. plain yogurt and
2 tbsp. sour cream

One cup of spaghetti or macaroni *or* two tablespoons of cooking oil (for sautéeing vegetables) are allowed any time you're willing to exchange them for the bread, saltines, yogurt and sour cream—remember, you must omit *all* these items.

Permitted: You may have up to four cups a day of any of the following *vegetables:*

brussels sprouts; broccoli; green or wax beans; cabbage; cauliflower; eggplant; kale; mung bean sprouts; mustard greens; mushrooms; spinach; turnips; turnip greens; zucchini

You may also partake of unlimited quantities of:

lettuce; celery; peppers; radishes; cucumbers; tomatoes; onions

You may have four servings per day of any of the following *fruits* (please note the size or amount specified; it constitutes a serving):

two fresh plums, peaches, nectarines or tangerines; half a fresh grapefruit or cantaloupe; one cup fresh watermelon or honeydew balls; one apple, orange or banana; one cup fresh cherries, blueberries, blackberries, strawberries or raspberries; one cup diced fresh pineapple

You may also have unlimited quantities of water, diet-free soda, black coffee or tea.

Not permitted: Any meat, poultry, fish, or eggs; and any food *not* specified in the VFD.

The Vegetable and Fruit Diet allows dieters to eat

quite a lot, and snacks—usually a piece of fruit—fit easily within the diet's framework. Following is a sample day's menu. Use your creativity to come up with your own interesting meal plans:

Breakfast: ⅓ cup strawberries, ⅓ cup blueberries, and ⅓ cup raspberries, topped with 5 tbsp. plain yogurt; 1 slice dry toast with 1 oz. melted cheddar cheese; black coffee or tea.

Mid-morning snack: One apple.

Lunch: ½ cup broccoli topped with 1 tbsp. sour cream; ½ cup carrots; ½ cup mushrooms; tossed green salad; 2 saltines; one tangerine; black coffee or tea.

Mid-afternoon snack: One peach.

Dinner: 1 cup sliced, broiled eggplant topped with 1 oz. Parmesan cheese; 1 cup stewed tomatoes; lettuce and tomato salad; 2 saltines; 1 cup diced fresh pineapple; black coffee or tea.

Late evening snack: One cup vegetable consommé.

Cooking tips: Learn to eat vegetables raw. Uncooked, they best retain natural vitamins and minerals, and you may even be surprised at how good they taste. Such unlikely candidates as broccoli, cauliflower and zucchini are marvelous when served raw and chilled. Dice these vegetables along with common salad ingredients, arrange them attractively on a platter or in a large bowl, chill and serve as hors d'oeuvres for parties or drinks. Or keep a bowl of cut-up raw vegetables (the French call it a *crudité*) in the refrigerator for between-meal nibbles. Prepare low-calorie yogurt or sour cream dips as accompaniment.

If you're cooking vegetables—which you most certainly will be doing on this diet—it's important to follow a few simple rules which will allow them to keep their nutrients and taste. Keep these four steps in mind when you're boiling vegetables:

1. Bring a small amount of (unsalted) water to boil.
2. Add vegetables and bring to second boil. Do not cover.
3. Reduce heat and simmer.
4. Remove vegetables before they are limp!

Season your vegetables with vinegar-mustard dressing, sour cream and/or herbs. Some natural go-together herbs are basil, bayleaf, cayenne pepper, chervil, curry powder, dill, marjoram, paprika, rosemary, sage, savory, tarragon and thyme. Stock a bare spice shelf with these items to enliven vegetarian dishes.

The Milk Diet

It was over 100 years ago that Dr. Philippe Karrell reduced his plump patients on menus of milk only; nearly 20 years ago that the Rockefeller Diet (milk mixed with sugar and corn oil) was *the* diet of its day; just 10 years ago that commercial milk-formula diets took the overweight society by storm. If you're a baby at heart—and who isn't—a creamy milk-base plan may be your smoothest path to sleek new shape.

The original milk diets called for three or four meals a day, all of them liquid, with no solids allowed. In recent years, however, the diet has been modified to permit one solid meal daily for those who wish it. The plan below is one of these modifications. Drink your breakfast and lunch, and chew your dinner!

THE MILK DIET MENUS

This regime totals 900 calories a day, over a third of them in the form of milk. If you follow the plan as outlined, you should shed between eight to 10 pounds in two weeks, and even more if you substitute skim milk when whole milk is called for.

Breakfast: Drink your milk like a good child: four ounces of whole milk combined with four ounces of skim. For variety, you may add cherry or vanilla extract, artificially sweetened chocolate syrup or other low-calorie sweetener.

Lunch: Exactly the same as breakfast: one eight-ounce glass of whole and skim milk.

Mid-afternoon snack: Again, for the third time, an eight-ounce drink of milk.

Dinner: For dinner, choose any lean cut of beef; one small baked or boiled potato; half a head of lettuce; and your choice of one cup spinach, cauliflower, carrots, cabbage or string beans.

Trim all visible fat from meat before cooking; broil or grill the meat without butter or other fat. Top your pristine potato with one tablespoon of chived sour cream; sprinkle herbed lemon juice or vinegar over your lettuce salad.

Cooking tips: Prepare delicious thick shakes by blending eight ounces of milk, several ice cubes, and your favorite flavoring in an electric blender. Mix for one minute to make a thick, creamy shake with no more calories than an ordinary glass of milk. Another flavoring tip: for coffee thick shakes, add ¼ cup of brewed black coffee to milk and ice. Blend together in an electric blender and serve immediately.

Diet hints: Sip milk through a straw. This child's method of drinking prevents you from gulping your milk, makes it last and last.

The Milk Diet has a marvelous side-effect, which I should mention: it's a natural tension-relaxer. Milk, the old-fashioned remedy for insomnia, is a rich source of calcium, which soothes the nerves as well as maintaining the health of the body's skeleton particularly the spine. Especially if you're a woman, you should continue to include milk, or an alternate calcium source, in your diet even after completing this diet. It will keep you standing straight and tall for the rest of your life!

The Eat-to-Lose-Weight Diet

New York City, home of Broadway and bright lights, Wall Street, fashionable department stores, the Statue of Liberty, fine restaurants and one of the smartest diets around today. It's called the Eat-to-Lose-Weight Diet, and let me tell you that you'll never feel the hint of a hunger pang or hear the rumble of a stomach as long as you follow this plan! Developed by the New York City Board of Nutrition for the overweight and the highly pressured, the Eat-to-Lose-Weight Diet allows you three substantial meals each day of your diet. A well-balanced, low-calorie regime, the ETLWD may be just your cup of tea if you want to lose weight, but don't want to change your eating patterns too, too drastically. In fact, this one's so simple to follow, you may hardly know you're dieting at all.

Do abide by the rules exactly, selecting foods from the "Food Facts" list that follows according to the diet's specific instructions. Vary your meals from day to day, and you'll have no trouble keeping to your diet—it's one of the super plans, as far as *this* dieter is concerned!

THE EAT-TO-LOSE-WEIGHT DIET MENUS

Breakfast
High Vitamin C Fruit
  Choose ONE from "Food Facts" on page 78
Protein Food—Choose ONE
  2 oz. cottage or pot cheese
  1 oz. hard cheese
  2 oz. cooked or canned fish
  1 egg
  8 oz. cup skimmed milk
Bread or Cereal, whole grain or enriched—Choose ONE
  1 slice bread
  ¾ cup ready-to-eat cereal
  ½ cup cooked cereal
Coffee or Tea

Lunch
Protein Food—Choose ONE
  2 oz. fish, poultry or lean meat
  4 oz. cottage or pot cheese
  2 oz. hard cheese
  1 egg
  2 level tablespoons peanut butter
Bread—whole grain or enriched—2 slices
Vegetables—raw or cooked—except potato or substitute
Coffee or Tea

Dinner

Protein Food—Choose ONE
    4 oz. cooked fish, poultry or lean meat
Vegetables cooked and raw
    High Vitamin A—Choose from "Food Facts"
    Potato or Substitute—Choose ONE from "Food Facts"
    Other Vegetables—you may eat freely
Fruit—1 serving
Coffee or Tea

Other Daily Foods

Fat—Choose 3 from "Food Facts"
Milk—2 cups (8 oz. each) skimmed or substitute from "Food Facts"

FOOD FACTS

Limit these protein foods
Lean beef, pork, lamb to
    1 lb. per week total
Eggs to 4 per week
Hard cheese to 4 oz. per week

High vitamin C fruits (no added sugar)

1 medium orange
½ medium cantaloupe
1 cup strawberries
½ medium mango
4 oz. orange or grapefruit juice
½ medium grapefruit
1 large tangerine
8 oz. tomato juice

Other fruits (no added sugar)

1 medium apple or peach
1 small banana or pear
¼ lb. cherries or grapes
½ cup pineapple
½ cup berries
2–3 apricots, prunes or plums
½ round slice watermelon (1" by 10")
½ small honeydew melon
2 tbsp. raisins

High vitamin A vegetables

broccoli
carrots
chicory
mustard greens, collards and other leafy greens
pumpkin, winter squash
spinach
watercress
escarole

Potato or substitute
1 medium potato
1 small sweet potato or yam
1 small ear corn
½ cup corn or green lima beans, peas
½ cup cooked dry beans, peas, lentils
½ cup cooked rice, spaghetti, macaroni, grits or noodles

Fat
1 tsp. vegetable oil
1 tsp. mayonnaise
2 tsp. French dressing
1 tsp. margarine with liquid vegetable oil noted first on ingredients label

Skim milk or substitute
2 cups (8 oz. each) buttermilk
1 cup (8 oz.) evaporated skimmed milk
⅔ cup nonfat dry milk solids

Beverages permitted
Coffee, tea, water, club soda, bouillon, consommé

Seasonings permitted
salt, pepper, herbs, spices, horscradish, lemon, lime, vinegar

Vegetables permitted (unlimited quantities)

asparagus	kale
green beans	lettuce
broccoli	mushrooms
brussels sprouts	mustard greens
carrots	parsley
cauliflower	romaine lettuce
celery	spinach
chicory	summer squash
collards	Swiss chard
cucumber	tomato
dandelion greens	turnip greens
escarole	watercress

Not permitted

bacon, fatty meats, sausage	gelatin desserts, puddings (sugar-sweetened)
beer, liquor, wines	gravies and sauces
butter, margarines other than described in	honey, jams, jellies, sugar and syrup

"Food Facts"

cakes, cookies, crackers, doughnuts, pastries, pies

candy, chocolates, nuts

cream—sweet and sour cream cheese, non-dairy cream substitutes

French-fried potatoes, potato chips

pizza, popcorn, pretzels and other snack foods

ice cream, ices, ice milk, sherbets

milk, whole

muffins, pancakes, waffles

olives

soda (sugar-sweetened)

yogurt (fruit-flavored)

Eat-to-Lose-Weight Dieters are very often over-weights the scale's caught up with; in other words, people who must lose upwards of 20 pounds. The diet lends itself particularly well to their special needs because of its slow, steady pace. On this 1200-calorie-per-day plan, average loss is two pounds per week—and a dieter may stay on it safely until every last pound is shed. For faster results, you could follow one of the Crash Diets (they're described beginning on page 119) for a week, and then switch over to the ETLWD—seeing the scale plummet by five pounds in almost as many days is the push most of us need to get us really going! Remember, crash diets are one-week-only plans. Consider the Eat-to-Lose-Weight Diet as your long-range regime.

The Champagne Diet

Has there ever been a more luxurious way to shed pounds than the Champagne Diet? *Vogue* printed this rich-girl pounds-off plan in October 1963, and it's been attracting glamorous slimmers ever since. To its many enthusiasts, sipping three goblets of sparkling champagne each day takes all the drudge out of dieting, making weight loss almost sport for anyone who likes to feel beautifully pampered.

But, good news! You don't have to be a jet-setter to follow the champagne bubbles; anyone can do it and expect to lose approximately three pounds per week. This is a low-cal plan that "offers joie de diet as well."

According to *Vogue,* you diet for seven days, but with each meal for each of these days—including breakfast and lunch as well as dinner—you drink one four-ounce glass of champagne. You can enjoy three lovely champagne glasses . . . Meals must be slimming ones; you should keep calories to under 1000 per day.

Vogue printed these sample menus for the champagne slimmer, but you should give your imagination free reign to create elegant diet meals worthy of this festive bubbling wine.

THE CHAMPAGNE DIET MENUS

Breakfast
½ cup orange juice
1 egg, scrambled in a double boiler
1 slice whole wheat toast
1 glass champagne

Lunch
mixed green salad
1 slice cold salmon
bran muffin
½ cantaloupe
1 glass champagne

Dinner
4 oz. broiled fillet of beef
cooked carrots
celery stalks
⅔ cup fresh strawberries
1 glass champagne

Breakfast
½ grapefruit
1 poached egg
1 small cinammon bun
1 glass champagne

Lunch
⅓ cup fruit cocktail
¾ cup crabmeat on a lettuce leaf
small French roll
1 glass champagne

Dinner
½ pear with cottage cheese
2 medium slices roast tenderloin of beef
cooked asparagus
carrot sticks
1 glass champagne

Unless otherwise indicated, all servings are half-cupfuls. You should garnish salads with a squeeze of lemon juice or a dash of wine vinegar; other dressings are too dear on this diet. It goes without saying that any meat you eat should be lean, with all visible fat trimmed off; and bread or buns must be eaten without butter or margarine.

Here are some of the meals I usually prepare while on the Champagne Diet. They're all easy to do, but just the same, make a dieter feel fabulous!

Breakfast
1 cup tomato juice
1 tsp. caviar and 2 tbsp. cottage cheese
2 slices melba toast
1 glass champagne

Breakfast
½ cup orange juice
½ cup broiled mushrooms on slice whole wheat toast
1 glass champagne

Lunch
1 cup chef's salad
3 bread sticks
1 glass champagne

Lunch
1 cup Waldorf salad
1 luncheon roll
1 glass champagne

Dinner
½ broiled grapefruit
4 oz. steak tartare (raw ground sirloin with herbs and seasoning)
spinach salad
1 glass champagne

Dinner
tossed green salad
scallops en brochette (broiled on skewers with bacon strips)
1 scoop raspberry ice
1 glass champagne

Use your own imagination to prepare luxurious, thinning meals. If you're not the world's most experienced chef, buy a good cookbook to give you some fresh ideas.

Diet hints: Unfortunately, champagne goes flat if left for any length of time—it should be sipped immediately after the cork is popped. Lessen the problem by buying miniature bottles, either imported or domestic, which contain smaller amounts of the bubbly. Store them in the refrigerator so that they're perfectly chilled when you're ready to dine.

Let me suggest, too, that this diet is one that automatically makes you focus on your looks—maybe because it's just so glamorous! Use your diet time to begin thinking about your appearance: hair, complexion and

wardrobe. Treat yourself to a day at the beauty
salon for a cut, wash and set, or if you're unhappy with
your current coif, get your crowning glory re-styled.
Ask the shampoo person for a hair conditioning treatment, too. A manicure and pedicure always make me
feel very well taken care of, and if you can afford these
niceties, they're a great morale booster. Pick up a few of
the fashion magazines—*Vogue, Harper's Bazaar, Ma-
demoiselle*—and leaf through the clothes-filled pages.
Notice new fashion trends. Try to develop a new interest by picking out the outfits you'd like to wear. I've
noticed that when I'm overweight I carefully avoid the
subject of clothes—sour grapes, I guess. It's never too
soon to change your outlook. Slimming down makes it
possible for all of us to look attractive and fashionable
in all the chicest new fashions! Remember, a slim new
figure is just weeks away.

THE LOW-CARBOHYDRATE DIETS

Call it "The Drinking Man's Diet," "The High-
Protein Diet," "The Eat All You Want Diet" or "The
Super Diet," this plan by any other name would still be
basically and beautifully the same: a reducing diet that
lets you eat your way to thinness by limiting carbohydrates while allowing you all the pure protein you want.
Choose a low-carb diet, and these usually forbidden
foods appear on your daily "yes" list: bacon, pork
chops, butter, hollandaise, sweet cream, a martini before dinner. Not bad for a diet, huh? Opt to go the low-
carbohydrate route and you can forget gnawing hunger
pangs; they just don't happen. Chuck out your calorie
counter, too: the only thing you have to watch is carbohydrate grams, and it's a breeze after having to nit-
pick each last food calorie on strict low-calorie regimes.
Friends of mine have even reported that low-carb dieting is almost like not dieting at all. And, what's more
important, these plans really work.
What's the magic behind low-carbohydrate dieting?
No magic, just a few simple rules which, when followed,
yield exciting results. Carbohydrates, as you know by

now, are starches and sugars, and that's what you must strenuously avoid for the duration of your diet. If you undertake one of these regimes, best be prepared to wave goodbye to bread, crackers, potatoes, pasta, rice, fruit and juices, candy, pastry, preserves, even sweetened cough drops.

That's the bad news. The good news, however, makes such taboos bearable, for you may, on most low-carbohydrate diets, eat unlimited amounts of pure protein. Mountains of steak, miles of roast beef, bushel baskets of poultry, fish and seafood, whatever your fancy desires. And since you're also permitted fats, you can douse salad greens with mayonnaise or drench your lobster tails in hot butter.

As I've already mentioned, low-carbohydrate dieting has been a recognized means of taking weight off for over a century. Until fairly recently, though, this method was relatively unknown, and most people who needed to lose simply counted calories. Now the tide has turned, and low-carbohydrate diets are in greater favor now than ever before. One important reason for this new popularity is the discovery by large numbers of chronically fat people that, astonishingly, counting carb grams actually causes weight loss. Thanks to low-carb diets, many chronic fatties are actually thin for the first time in their lives. I can assure you that a diet which focuses on stick-to-the-ribs proteins and fats is a blessing to anyone who gains weight at the drop of a cookie. No small consideration for those who could formerly lose only via starvation methods.

The theory behind low-carb dieting is that the main culprit in excess flab is carbohydrates—those nasty starches and sugars. For people who burn carbohydrates at an abnormal rate, limiting these "danger" foods facilitates weight loss. Even for those with more even body chemistries, low-carbohydrate dieting is a painless way to slim. This is why: on any of these plans, you consume generous portions of food. You also eat to the point of fullness. Because protein and fat foods take longer to digest than carbohydrates, you won't experience hunger, irritability or temptation.

The diets in this section are classics. Tried and tested

by millions, these low-carb plans will help you to drop every last unwanted pound. The most popular variations of the diet fall into two categories: the low-carbohydrate and the ultra-low-carbohydrate. What makes the two different is that the low-carb plans allow servings of fruits and vegetables, while the ultra-low ones don't. If, after reading through all the diets, you decide you'd like to try a controlled carbohydrate diet, choose the one most appealing to your palate and to your imagination. Follow the directions to the minute. Do not—I repeat, do *not*—switch back and forth from a low-carb to a low-calorie diet. If you do, neither will work and, what's worse, you'll probably gain weight. Again, a medical check-up and your doctor's go-ahead are strongly suggested before you take the low-carbohydrate leap—or, for that matter, before you begin *any* diet.

The 10-Day-10-Pounds-Off Diet

Lose a pound a day for 10 days on this sunshine low-carb plan. Ever since it appeared in *Cosmopolitan* in September 1970, this has been one of my all-time favorite diets because it's super-easy as well as effective. Unlike most other plans, it permits fruit—delicious, tangy grapefruit—three times a day. Some nutritionists believe that grapefruit may act as a catalyst in burning body fat, but for me, it serves a more important purpose: it satisfies the craving most low-carb dieters get for fruit, and for anything that's sweet. Grapefruit's natural sugars give you a taste of both.

The 10-Day-10-Pounds-Off Diet caused a furor when it first appeared in the London *Times* during the summer of 1970. According to *Cosmo,* London *Times'* women's editor Ernestine Carter introduced the new diet that had enabled fashion designer John Cavanagh to shed the unwelcome weight he put on after quitting smoking, and finished her column with the innocent invitation to readers to try this "friendly, neighborhood, nearly infallible diet" by sending a stamped, self-addressed envelope to her in care of the paper. Then

4000 replies poured in, after just two days! And that
didn't include the countless phone requests that jammed
the *Times'* switchboard for days afterward. From London, the diet spread to France and Holland, and *Cosmo*
reports that it's been burning off fat successfully ever
since.

The basics of the diet couldn't be easier, but you
must stick exactly to the rules. The diet's success relies
on the proper balancing of foods, so if you cheat by so
much as a slice of chewing gum, you're throwing the
balance off kilter. You won't reduce; in fact, you might
see your scale shoot up instead. Be vigilant!

THE 10-DAY-10-POUNDS-OFF MENUS

Here's what you can and can't eat on this low-carb
plan. I'll begin with the foods allowed on your daily
menus and I can tell you in advance that each diet day
is a joy. The pounds will seem to melt away while
you're enjoying delicious protein-packed meals.

Breakfast: If you're the slightest bit tempted to cheat
the night before, just picture next morning's hearty
breakfast menu. You may have:

     ½ grapefruit or
     6 oz. unsweetened grapefruit juice

     eggs, up to 12, cooked any style
     bacon slices, as many as 12

     1 cup black coffee or plain tea

There's one rule you must adhere to, and that is to
eat an equal number of eggs and bacon slices, but not
more than a dozen (I have never known anyone who
felt limited by this particular restriction)! So, if you
have four eggs, you must have four slices of bacon, and
vice versa. Note, too, that only one cup of black coffee
or plain tea is permitted.

Lunch: Lunch is a feast, so sit down at the table and
prepare to enjoy. The menu is as follows:

½ grapefruit or
6 oz. unsweetened grapefruit juice

unlimited quantity of meat

tossed green salad

black coffee or plain tea

Begin this meal, as you will every meal, with grape-fruit. Your entree consists of as much pure meat as you wish; you may fry, boil, bake or broil meat with any amount of butter, and serve any meat juice that runs off as gravy. There are no stops on the salad, either; eat as much as you please. Top salad with olive oil and vine-gar dressing. Remember, only one cup of black coffee or plain tea—as if you'd have room for a second.

Though the basic luncheon menu is the same throughout all 10 days of the diet, you can easily vary meals with different choices of meat and different meth-ods of preparation. I've been on the diet twice, and here are some of the entrees I enjoyed most at noon:

cold, baked or boiled ham slices
frankfurters, grilled in butter
cold roast beef or lamb slices
ground beef, sautéed in butter

These are tasty meals, and filling ones, too, a breeze to whip up at home or enjoy in just about any kind of restaurant.

Dinner: Dinner is a repeat of lunch, with one excep-tion: you may, in addition to the regular menu, have as much as you wish of any "permitted" vegetables from the list below.

½ grapefruit or
6 oz. unsweetened grapefruit juice

unlimited quantity of meat

unlimited quantities of "permitted" vegetables

tossed salad

black coffee or plain tea

Feel free to top the vegetables with butter—liberally. Or, live it up with a creamy butter-made hollandaise sauce.

The second time on this diet, I finally got to feeling that I couldn't face another piece of unadorned meat. If you reach that same point, break the steak-and-chops pattern with a few entrees like these:

> short ribs of beef braised with 3 oz. dry red wine
>
> veal cutlets, sautéed in butter then simmered with 2 oz. dry vermouth
>
> beef tenderloin, broiled and basted with melted butter and 1 oz. brandy

Permitted: Permitted vegetables on the 10-Day plan are all the non-starchy, non-sweet varieties. You can forget about potatoes, corn, peas and beans. Concentrate on thinning . . .

> asparagus, broccoli, brussels sprouts, cabbage, cauliflower, collards, escarole, kale, mustard greens, parsley, spinach, turnip greens, watercress

Any kind of lettuce—romaine, bibb, Boston, etc.—may be used in salad-making along with unlimited quantities of cucumber, celery and tomato.

You may not use margarine on this diet; you must use butter, but you can have as much butter as you like. Use olive, vegetable, peanut, soy or safflower oil with vinegar for salad dressings.

One of the loveliest things about the 10-Day plan is that the dieter is allowed wine and liquor. Use them in cooking or for imbibing or both. Drinks may be served on the rocks or with water or soda. I don't recommend lots of guzzling, but I'll tell you that I enjoyed a nightly drink before dinner and lost all 10 pounds on schedule.

Diet hints: Weigh yourself when you start on the plan, but resist the temptation to check your progress until the fifth day. Why wait so long? Because an oddity of this diet is that the scale doesn't surrender an ounce for the first four days. Your reward comes on the morning of the fifth day: you should be five pounds lighter—and every day thereafter you should lose another pound. Ten days of dieting; 10 pounds off!

Dr. Atkins' Diet Revolution

Dr. Robert Atkins, the famous obesity specialist who designed this rapid weight-loss system, calls his diet a "revolution," and you may, too, if you've run the gamut of low-calorie plans without much success. On Dr. Atkins' Diet you can eat as much as you want, as often as you want; you can eat heretofore prohibited foods— steak, butter, cream, cheese, mayonnaise and other rich foods; and, you'll lose tons of weight—for most people, five to 10 pounds the first week and two to five pounds per week after that!

Dr. Atkins' weight-loss theory (yes, it's controversial) holds carbohydrates totally responsible for our national fat problems, and sternly prohibits those "bad guy" sugars and starches altogether for the first leg of the diet. During the second week, you're allowed to add a few carbohydrates, during the third week just a few more—but if you stick with this eating plan (and Dr. Atkins would have you stay with it for life!), you'll never be able to eat very *many* carbohydrates. No, the focus of the Atkins Diet is proteins and fats, permitted in inexhaustible quantities. Eat all you want; you'll lose weight and never feel hungry on this program.

Originally published in *Vogue* magazine in 1970, where it was billed as the "Super Diet," Atkins' plan was a 16-day regime for those who wanted to lose 10–12 pounds. The Diet Revolution, which I describe here, is slightly revised and aimed more for anyone who wants to lose upwards of 10 pounds. But, you can still follow it, no matter how much you plan to lose. If you have less to lose, stay on each diet "level" for four days; if you have more to lose, remain on each level for one week.

If the Atkins' Diet works as well for you as it has for others, you may want the book *Dr. Atkins' Diet Revo-*

lution (McKay, hardcover; Bantam, paperback) in which the doctor discusses how you can adjust your low-carb diet for a lifetime maintenance program. Dr. Atkins suggests—and I heartily concur—that you have a medical check-up before beginning this diet. Discuss the diet with your own doctor, and see what he has to say about it for you. If you get an OK, join the thousands of dieters who have already made this plan a diet classic.

DR. ATKINS' DIET REVOLUTION MENUS

Your choice of foods on the Atkins' Diet is wide (wider, for example, than the choice offered on the 10-Day-10-Pounds-Off Diet). However, before I get to the menus, it's important to note these basic rules:

1. Take a multivitamin pill every day. The so-called therapeutic tablets or capsules are best, since they have a higher vitamin-mineral content than simple once-daily vitamins.

2. Prevent hunger by eating frequently. Six small meals a day are preferable to three large ones, but if you're really not hungry—don't eat at all. Learn to differentiate between appetite, which is the *desire* to eat, and hunger, which is the *need* to eat.

3. Watch out for "unseen carbohydrates." Sugar is present even in many so-called "diet" products, so read the labels on packaged and canned foods carefully before you buy, and run, run, run from anything containing either sugar or starch.

4. Drink as much water as you like, though you need not force yourself. Calorie-free soda and other sugarless fluids are also permitted in unlimited quantities. Limit your intake of regular coffee to no more than four cups a day; fewer if you can. If you're a coffee addict, switch over after the fourth cup to a decaffeinated brand and then drink to your heart's content.

The Atkins' Diet has five basic phases. Food is most strictly limited in the first phase, but the rules ease up as you go along, and additional foods may be included. In other words, this diet has its own built-in incentive;

the longer you stick with it, the more delicious items are added to your "yes" list.

LEVEL ONE: Only the following foods are permitted for the initial phase of your diet. Eat all you need to satisfy hunger. Eat again when you get hungry. Here's the OK list:

Pure meat: Unlimited quantities of any kind of pure meat, including pork; you may *not* have luncheon meat, sausage, non-beef hot dogs or any type of meat which is mixed with other ingredients. Be leery about ordering hamburger, meatloaf and similar entrees when you eat out. Even fine restaurants sometimes stretch chopped beef by adding bread crumbs or cracker meal.

Poultry: Unlimited quantities of poultry, including game birds, are permitted; choose white meat or dark. If you're bored with chicken or turkey, ask the butcher to order pheasant, squab or even a pair of quail!

Fish and seafood: Most varieties are allowed in unlimited amounts, with these exceptions: no clams, oysters, mussels or scallops. You may have fish packed in oil—tuna and sardines, for example—and smoked fish like Nova Scotia salmon, sturgeon, sable, whitefish, etc. All in unlimited quantities.

Cheese: Only hard, aged cheese is permitted, and you must limit yourself to four ounces per day. Consider Swiss, cheddar, Roquefort, gorgonzola, and Parmesan cheeses. Soft and semi-soft cheeses are not allowed; neither are cheese spreads and cheese foods, such as cottage cheese or cream cheese.

Eggs: As many as you want per day, cooked any way you want. The only restriction is that you may not use milk in their preparation.

Salad: You may have two small green salads per day, each less than one cupful, loosely packed. You may *not* have more salad than this. Prepare salad using lettuce, cucumber, celery, radishes, onion, peppers or pimiento. No tomatoes! Dress your salad with oil and vinegar or, if you prefer, a dollop of real mayonnaise.

Fats and oils: You are allowed as much butter, margarine, shortening or other oils as you wish; remember, though, that you'll lose quicker if you don't go crazy with butter and oil; deep-frying everything, for example, isn't recommended.

Heavy cream: You are allowed four teaspoons of heavy cream a day. Note that you may *not* substitute milk (as in coffee, for example). You must have the cream or nothing at all.

Seasonings and condiments: Artificial sweeteners and flavor extracts such as vanilla, rum and peppermint; any spices that contain no sugar, such as salt, pepper, garlic powder, garlic salt, onion flakes, onion salt, thyme, marjoram and tarragon. By the way, Dr. Atkins recommends salting food liberally while on the diet to make up for the natural salt depletion that happens with dieting. The permitted condiments are limited to mustard, mayonnaise, vinegar, horseradish and the juice of one lemon or lime.

Dessert: Unflavored or artificially sweetened gelatin is approved for dessert. Add flavor extracts, such as peppermint, to the unflavored kind for a delicious after-dinner treat.

Beverages: Of course, you may have unlimited glass-fuls of water, diet soda, decaffeinated coffee and tea. Broth and bouillon in either beef or chicken flavor are permitted. I would recommend the cube or packet types, with lower-carbohydrate content than canned broths. To add pick-me-up flavor, sprinkle broth and bouillon with finely-chopped scallions.

Stay at Level One for one week (or four days if you have less to lose). You should notice the pounds melting away.

LEVEL TWO: Beginning the second week of your diet, you may add approximately five to eight carbohydrate grams daily to your menu. Put back the food that you've missed most—but only five grams worth! You must have a carbohydrate gram counter and a gram scale (both widely sold) in order to be accurate about your carbos.

Here is what Dr. Atkins suggests adding. He says that most of his patients add cottage cheese at Level

Two, or cottage cheese and another food. It doesn't matter, so long as you don't exceed eight carbohydrate grams per day. Certain kinds of nuts (walnuts, pecans, Brazils and macadamias) are surprisingly low in carbohydrates and you may choose them to snack on during the day. Or a bit of tomato or onion for cooking is preferable to some dieters. Count your carbo grams—you must if you're going to keep the pounds rolling off.

LEVEL THREE: OK. You've been on the diet for two weeks and should have lost approximately nine or 10 pounds. Beginning the third week, you may add another five to eight carbohydrate grams daily to your ration. Dr. Atkins recommends the addition of vegetables here, to make life a bit more interesting. Following his suggestion, you may have one-half cup, or one small serving, of these low-gram vegetables: asparagus, avocado, bamboo shoots, bean sprouts, broccoli, brussels sprouts, cabbage, cauliflower, eggplant, kale, mushrooms, okra, onions, peppers, rhubarb, sauerkraut, snow pea pods, spinach, string beans, tomatoes, turnips, wax beans and zucchini. Remember, this vegetable allowance (or whatever food you choose to add) is *in addition* to the five to eight grams you added at Level Two, making a total allowance of between 10 to 16 carbohydrate grams daily.

LEVEL FOUR: Add another five to eight grams here, bringing your daily limit to between 15 and 24 carbo grams per day (of course, the fewer grams you add, the more rapid your weight loss).

At this level, Dr. Atkins permits dieters to have alcohol; for example, one glass of dry red or white wine. Since alcohol is gram-expensive, you must be vigilant. Atkins recommends that you have no more than four ounces of scotch or whiskey weekly; or three ounces of scotch or whiskey *and* a small glass of wine or champagne.

At Level Four, many dieters choose to add fruit; for instance, cantaloupe or berries or a half-grapefruit twice a week. Be sure to check carefully the carbohydrate contents of fruits; they're invariably high, and exceeding your limit will only impede your weight loss.

LEVEL FIVE: Add another five to eight grams, bringing you to between 20 and 29 carbohydrate grams daily. Some friends of mine have said that here they've added bread—one slice of any regular bread or two slices of gluten bread; I myself have juggled grams in order to have ¼ cup of ice cream (10 gms.) or else, simply added one cup of skim milk (3.8 gms.). Work it out for yourself with the foods you've been missing.

If, after five weeks and five levels of the Atkins' Diet, you are still overweight, continue on the diet, adding between five to eight grams of carbohydrate each week. Stay on the diet until you're down to your desired weight. As you approach the finish line, your loss should be at the rate of approximately a pound a week.

How to use Ketostix: Dr. Atkins recommends using Ketostix to check the progress of your diet each day. These testing sticks, available without prescription in drug stores and pharmacies, test your urine for ketones, which are the waste products formed when actual fat is burned in the body. When ketones are present in the urine, the Ketostix turn purple. This is desirable, according to Dr. Atkins. He suggests testing each day; after about four days on the diet, the sticks should be purple. Thereafter, they should be purple each day. If they seem pale in color, first check that you are following the diet exactly. If you have followed instructions to the tee, then cut back on your carbohydrate intake until the Ketostix show up purple again. This is very fully explained in Dr. Atkins' book, should you wish to know more about it.

DR. ATKINS' DIET REVOLUTION MENUS

Meals can be delicious and interesting on the Atkins' Diet, even within the framework of Level One! Here are some menus I've enjoyed on this diet. This diet is flexible enough so that I never once felt the desire to cheat. If you do, just slap your wrists, and walk away from temptation.

Level One

Breakfast: Small minute steak; fried eggs; coffee with cream.

Lunch: Boiled flounder topped with butter and Parmesan cheese; ½ cup leafy green salad with mayonnaise dressing; coffee with cream.

Dinner: Pure-beef frankfurters, split lengthwise and grilled with cheddar cheese; leafy green salad with sesame seeds, oil and vinegar dressing; diet cola.

Level Two

Breakfast: Cheese omelette; 2 tomato wedges; coffee with cream.

Lunch: Salad platter, including: one can tuna fish; ½ cup cottage cheese; 3 asparagus spears; scallions; radish florets, all on a bed of lettuce; iced tea.

Dinner: Cucumber and pimiento salad, seasoned with pepper, oil, vinegar and chopped chervil; 2 medium loin lamb chops; almond-flavored gelatin dessert. Coffee with cream.

Level Three

Breakfast: Cottage cheese (½ cup); Nova Scotia salmon; cucumber slices; 4 slim tomato wedges; celery stalks; black coffee.

Lunch: Deviled eggs; tossed green salad with oil and vinegar dressing; glass of dry white wine.

Dinner: Consommé; chicken breasts with mushroom sauce; asparagus tips with butter; braised lettuce; 6 strawberries topped with cream; coffee.

Level Four

Breakfast: Scrambled eggs with bacon slices; coffee with cream.

Lunch: ¼ lb. boiled shrimp, chilled; escarole salad with Roquefort dressing; iced tea with lemon.

Dinner: Steak with wine and mushroom sauce; sautéed brussels sprouts with parsley; pickled cucumber salad; coffee with cream.

Cooking tips: Now is a good time to invest in a diet cookbook, preferably one that lists carbohydrate con-

tents for each recipe dish. So many interesting meals are
possible on the Atkins' Diet, you'll be able to polish
your culinary skills while shedding pounds. Be experimental. Use this diet as an opportunity to learn something new about the food you eat: different kinds of
food, different styles of cooking, different ways of serving. Remember, food is only as exciting as the cook
who prepares it!

Diet hints: The Atkins' Diet is a sociable diet. You
can entertain while you're on it, and you don't have to
be afraid of dinners out. Simply shake your head "no"
to all sugars and starches, even if everyone else is oooh-
ing and aaahing over a particularly scrumptious-looking
dish. In fact, I find it useful to dine out with friends
because it takes away that awful feeling of being sen-
tenced to solitary confinement. Just follow the rules
(even if you have to carry them around with you on a
slip of paper) and let your friends marvel at how you
can eat so much and still be losing so much weight.

One general piece of advice for any dieter seems per-
tinent here. You don't have to finish everything on your
plate. "Licking the platter clean" is most often a vestige
from childhood when Mother urged you to join the
ranks of children who were "good eaters." Break that
habit, which often forces you to eat more than you
might really want, by leaving a bit of food on your
plate, even the tiniest morsel. This act will teach you—
eventually, anyway—to be sensitive to your own hunger.

If, by any chance, you should experience tiredness or
a washed-out feeling on the Atkins' Diet, do one of two
things: first, try increasing your intake of salt. If you
still feel logy, add more carbohydrates to your intake,
just enough to allow you to feel bright and energetic.

One of the outstanding features of the Atkins' Diet is
the enthusiasm it generates among those who have gone
on it. Try it. You may even love it, too.

The Drinking Man's Diet

You don't have to be an out-and-out lush to enjoy this low-carbohydrate diet, but if you do like a drink or a glass of wine now and again, this may be the perfect plan for you. You can lose between 10 and 15 pounds in a month, and still enjoy your nightly cocktail, too. Pure distilled liquor (rum, scotch, vodka, gin, whiskey,) contains only a trace of carbo grams. Therefore, you may include as *many* drinks as you can handle—but have them without gram-rich additives.

Also known as the Air Force Diet (after the Air Force Academy where it was rumored to have been invented), the Drinking Man's Diet burst on the scene in 1964, and it's as popular today as it was a decade ago. Though the Air Force has disowned the diet, millions have adopted it with enormous success. As well as allowing alcoholic beverages, this plan was the first one to place *no* restrictions on what you eat.

Well, to be perfectly accurate, almost no restrictions. On the DMD, you may eat anything you like so long as your daily intake of starches and sugars does not exceed 60 carbohydrate grams.

And what's a carbohydrate gram? It is simply a measure of the amount of carbohydrate present in a particular food. On a calorie diet, you count calories; here, you count carbohydrate grams, limiting the total consumed to under 60 per day. It's not difficult; in fact, for many dieters, gram-watching is much easier than calorie-counting.

All you need is a carbohydrate gram counter: and a generic one is provided for you on pages 197–288.

As I've said, you'll lose between 10 and 15 pounds per month if you're like most people. Of course, your loss will be greater and quicker if you limit your carbohydrate intake to average 45–50 grams a day.

You can eat *anything* with the Drinking Man's Diet as long as you limit yourself to no more than 60 carbohydrate grams per day. The meals you choose and the foods you opt to include are strictly a matter of personal preference. That's why two people, both following the DMD, might never eat the same meal! For individualists, gourmets and those with well-entrenched eating habits, this diet is like an answered prayer.

To get an idea of how much you can eat on a low-gram diet, bear in mind that the following foods contain zero carbohydrate grams.

pure beef	pure pork
pure lamb	pure poultry
pure veal	pure fish

(Note that "pure" simply means all meat, no fillers of any kind added; steak, for example, is pure beef. Organ meats such as liver, kidney, etc., are *not* zero-gram foods—their gram content must be calculated in your daily carbo total.)

And to see how varied this diet can be, bear in mind that these are just some of the foods that contain less than one carbohydrate gram.

3 eggs	3 oz. crab meat
2 tbsp. cream	3 oz. shrimp
1 oz. most cheeses	½ cup lobster meat
4 slices bacon	1 oz. caviar

More good news: butter and margarine have less than a single gram per whole half cup; two heaping tablespoons of real mayonnaise contain less than one gram; salad and cooking oils have no carbohydrates whatever.

Your gram counter is your best friend. As you become familiar with the gram weights of various carbohydrate foods, you will see that by planning meals carefully, you can stick to your diet, but occasionally splurge with "fattening" goodies forbidden on other low-carb plans. If, for example, you limit your daytime eating to low- or no-gram foods (meat, cheese, eggs, etc.), you can let loose in the evenings with starches and sugars such as a hamburger roll (20.9 grams), Jeno Jr. pepperoni pizza (23.8 grams), two medium tangerines (20 grams), a whole package of Stouffer's au gratin potatoes (35.6 grams), three beloved Mallomars (25.8 grams)—any of those delicious sugars and starches you find hardest to give up.

Below is a sample menu, where you will see how you can stay within the DMD rules and still enjoy a full-fledged Italian dinner if you limit your breakfast and lunch with super-low-carb foods.

> *Breakfast:* Half-cup tomato juice (5.2 grams); mushroom omelette, made with ¼ cup mushrooms (1.1 grams); 1 thin slice white toast with butter (8.6 grams); coffee or tea.
>
> *Lunch:* Highball, broiled chopped steak with a slice of Bermuda onion (1.5 grams); tossed green salad with 2 tbsp. blue cheese dressing (4.9 grams); iced tea.
>
> *Dinner:* Highball, tossed green salad with oil and vinegar dressing (3.0 grams); 8 oz. can cheese ravioli with sauce (30 grams); 3½ oz. glass Chianti (4.3 grams); espresso.

Total grams for the day: 59.2 carbohydrate grams! You're under the quota, and should be feeling absolutely satisfied.

Diet hints: There are surprising differences in the carbohydrate contents of the "same" kinds of brand-name foods. Why? It's obvious, if you just stop to think about it. Different companies use different recipes in making the same product, just as you and your neighbor might add your own distinctive flavorings to a chicken salad, for example. While you and she might both begin with chicken, eggs and mayonnaise, you might flavor your salad with green pepper and onion and she might prefer to add chopped walnuts and sweet pickles. If you eat a lot of commercially prepared foods (frozen or canned) I would suggest buying a brand-name carbohydrate counter, which lists products according to label as well as including the common types of food, generic items like fresh vegetables and fruits. Dell publishes *The Brand-Name Carbohydrate Gram Counter,* and other companies also put out brand-name counters in hardcover and paperback.

The Calories-Don't-Count Diet

Calories Don't Count was one of the diet best-sellers of the early 1960s. Developed by Dr. Herman Taller, a New York gynecologist and obstetrician, this low-carb plan was followed by thousands, with marvelously successful results. Although the "three ounces of safflower oil" per day originally prescribed by the diet has since been proved unnecessary to successful weight loss, the diet itself will help you take pounds and inches off quickly. If you don't like too much fuss in the kitchen, if you like your diets simple and straightforward, this American classic might be the perfect plan for you.

Permitted foods:
1. *Pure meats:* Trim off all visible fat before eating.
2. *Poultry*
3. *Fish and seafood:* All forms of seafood, with natural oils and fats.
4. *Eggs*
5. *Gluten bread:* This low-carbo product is the only type of bread permitted. (A recipe appears on page 150, if you want to make your own.)
6. *Vegetables:* Artichokes, asparagus, string beans, beet greens, broccoli, brussels sprouts, cabbage, cauliflower, celery, chard leaves, cucumber, eggplant, endive, escarole, kale, leek, lettuce, mushrooms, okra, green peppers, pumpkin, radishes, rhubarb, sauerkraut, spinach, summer squash, tomatoes, turnip, watercress. (Two 3 oz. servings permitted at lunch; two 3 oz. servings at dinner.)
7. *Fruits:* Avocado, muskmelon (cantaloupe or honeydew), watermelon.
8. *Shell nuts*
9. *Cheese:* All kinds of cheese.
10. *Milk:* Not more than one cup per day (taken by most dieters with coffee or tea).
11. *Butter, margarine, fats, oils*
12. *Artificially sweetened carbonated soft drinks*

13. *Coffee and tea:* With artificial sweeteners, no sugar.

You may eat as much as you want from the list above, but it is suggested by Dr. Taller that large amounts of meat, poultry, fish or seafood be consumed when you include them on your menu—a lunch or dinner protein portion should be at least six to eight ounces' worth!

Here are Dr. Taller's own guidelines for following the CDC Diet:

1. Eat three meals each day—don't skip any meals.
2. Eat until you are full, but don't stuff yourself.
3. Eat fish or seafood at least once a day.
4. Drink plenty of water—at least three glasses between breakfast and lunch, and three glasses between lunch and dinner.
5. Avoid dried foods.
6. Do not salt your food—use substitute herbs and seasonings.
7. Avoid alcohol.
8. Walk at least one hour each day.
9. Do not eat anything not on the permitted list. The following foods are to be avoided:

Not permitted: Fruits not on the "permitted" list; fruit juices; vegetables not on the "permitted" list; vegetable juices; breads, except for gluten bread; starches; sugars; cakes, cookies or pastries; candy and chocolate; ice cream and ices; light and heavy cream; any beverage containing sugar.

Don't expect fat that's accumulated over years to disappear overnight. Dr. Taller reminds us that this is not a *crash* program, and that weight loss might take weeks or months, depending on how many pounds you need to take off. You can speed up or retard the rate of loss by including fewer or more items from the carbohydrate list: to reduce super-fast, eat a minimum of carbohydrates—cut your consumption of gluten bread, vegetables, fruits, shell nuts and milk, while increasing the no-carbohydrate meats, poultry, fish and eggs.

Diet hints: You don't count calories on this plan; you don't count grams. Without such time-consuming

diversions, some dieters—I know I'm one of them—
find strict diet plans like the CDC Diet a trifle boring.
The way to combat boredom? Use your diet as a good
time to begin a new project. Redecorate a room, make
new slipcovers for your favorite chairs, take a course at
the local college, learn embroidery or bargello, anything
you like so long as your attention is yanked far, far
away from the kitchen (for this reason, as you might
guess, redecorating the kitchen isn't the best idea ever).
Take up a new hobby, if you've always suspected some
hidden talent: writing, painting, a musical instrument,
carpentry, pottery, weaving . . . the interest will stay
with you long after pounds are gone.

Dr. Stillman's Quick Weight-loss Diet

Is there anyone who doesn't know Dr. Irwin
("Stilly") Stillman, the Brooklyn doctor who rediscov-
ered water? Author of this decade's most popular diet,
the late Dr. Stillman taught over six million overweight
Americans how to shed unwanted pounds with a
weight-loss plan that includes over half a gallon of water a day! Converts to Dr. Stillman's gospel include the
rich and the famous: Carol Burnett, Barbra Streisand
and the Jackies, Onassis and Gleason. If you're looking
for a super-fast way to lose lots of weight, consider joining the ever-growing Stillman fan club. The emphasis of
his Quick Weight-loss Diet is speed.

Fat, said Dr. Stillman, is killing us by increasing
among Americans the incidence of coronary disease,
high blood pressure, diabetes and hardening of the arteries. What's the best insurance for a long and fruitful
life? Lose that flab!

His diet is an absolute marvel. If followed faithfully,
it can result in the loss of five to 10 percent of your
total body weight within the first week of dieting. Unlike most other low-carb programs, the QWLD permits
no fats whatever. It's an ultra-high protein diet that
curbs food allowances to the barest minimum in order
to hasten weight loss. I can vouch for this diet's results

myself; it helped me to lose 10 pounds in eight days at a time when I needed to get thin quickly.

THE QUICK WEIGHT-LOSS BASICS

If you're not good about sticking to the rules, this diet is not for you. Success requires unquestioning adherence to the plan, which is fairly strict. In particular, the water business (explained below) is important. You must drink each and every last ounce for this diet to work.

Comedienne Joan Rivers, another of Dr. Stillman's converts, once cracked that you can eat anything on the QWLD "that walks, swims or flies." As you'll see, the permitted foods on the diet can be summarized just about that simply. Essentially, the plan relies on five basic food items: meat, chicken, fish, eggs and cheese.

And, of course, water. *You must drink 80 ounces of water a day*. That means eight tall glasses or, if you prefer, 16 half glasses every day you stay on this diet. (For obvious reasons, this diet is also known as the Water Diet). According to Dr. Stillman, the purpose of such huge quantities of water is to wash waste products and ashes of burned fat from the body; in other words, to cleanse the system. And I will admit, that you do feel purged and internally immaculate after more than a half-gallon of water each day. I found that the most comfortable way to program my drinks was at hourly intervals: one eight-ounce cup of water every hour on the hour, for 10 hours. This practice became routine for me and after one day, no bother at all.

Dr. Stillman also recommends that dieters take a multi-vitamin supplement once a day, or twice a day if you're over 40 or plan to keep eating to a minimum. Choose a pill that contains vitamin A (5000 USP units), vitamin D (500 units), vitamin B-1 (3 mg.), vitamin B-2 (3 mg.), vitamin C (50 mg.) as well as other vitamins and minerals.

THE QUICK WEIGHT-LOSS FOODS

As I've mentioned, this is a bare-bones diet. The list of "permitted" foods is rather short and short on variety, too. Though you can invent interesting meals within the QWLD's guidelines, let me be frank in admitting that this is no gourmet eating plan. Meals are usually simple, quick to fix and basic. If you experience boredom, which some Stillman dieters do, be reassured that this feeling may be supplanted only by a decreasing interest in eating at all—which means that you'll lose weight even more quickly! You may eat as much as you want of the foods listed below. If you eat less, you'll drop weight faster. A good general rule is to eat until you are full. Eat again only when you are hungry. And don't ever stuff yourself.

Here's the list. Again, these foods are allowed in unlimited quantities:

Permitted:
Meat: You may have any pure lean meat, except pork, ham, bacon and organ meats—liver, kidneys, brains, sweetbreads. Luncheon meats like salami and bologna are *not* permitted. Meat should be cooked by broiling, boiling or roasting, and all visible fat must be trimmed before eating. Frying is not an acceptable cooking method on the QWLD.

Chicken or turkey: Other fatty poultry—duck, goose and Rock Cornish game hen, for example, are *not* allowed. Prepare chicken or turkey by boiling, broiling, roasting or baking. Make sure to remove skin before eating.

Fish: All varieties of fish are permitted, with the exception of smoked, salted or pickled fish. Canned tuna and salmon are fine, so long as they are water-packed.

Shellfish: Enjoy many types of seafood including lobster tails, prawns and crab legs. You may *not* fry shellfish; rather, prepare by broiling, boiling or poaching. Since butter, margarine and oils are not permitted on this diet, substitute herbs, spices and other seasonings to add flavor in cooking.

Skim-milk cheeses: Look for 100% skim milk cheeses; some cheeses, labeled "partially-skim milk" contain whole milk, which is not allowed on this plan.

Cottage cheese: You may also have pot cheese and farmer cheese. Cottage cheese mixed with pineapple or garden vegetables is *not* permitted.

Eggs: Serve eggs either boiled or poached, and if your cholesterol level is high, limit your intake to four eggs per week.

Bouillon: Bouillon, broth or consommé, beef or chicken, are permitted—but *not* the canned varieties.

Club soda: You may drink unlimited quantities of club soda or other sugar-free soft drink. These beverages, however, are not to be considered as substitutes for water; however many soft drinks you have, you must still include your eight daily glasses of water.

Gelatin: Sugar-free gelatin is allowed on this diet.

Coffee and tea: Although Dr. Stillman doesn't say so, I would recommend limiting yourself to three cups of coffee or tea per day—more than this amount tends to make people on this diet jittery. Decaffeinated coffee is highly recommended for this reason. Note again that coffee and tea do *not* replace your water requirement.

Seasonings and condiments: You may have unlimited salt, pepper, vinegar, garlic, onion powder, tabasco and dried herbs. The following condiments should be taken in moderation: catsup, chili sauce, cocktail sauce, mustard, horseradish and relish.

Artificial sweeteners: Since no sugar is allowed on this program, sweeten beverages and gelatin with a sugar substitute.

That's the list. Only these foods are permitted on this ultra-high-protein diet. The diet's a radical one, truly, so it's very important that you check in with your doctor before beginning it. If he gives you the green light, begin your diet with a solemn vow to eat only the food items printed on the preceding list.

I think it's important to include also the foods that are *not* permitted on the Stillman Water Diet. Most of them are so ingrained in our eating patterns that dieters often have to be reminded that these familiar items must be locked away for the duration of this diet.

Not permitted:

Liquor, wine, beer or other alcoholic beverages	Vegetables
	Vegetable juices
Sugar	Fruits
Sweets	Fruit juices
Fats	Smoked fish
Butter, margarine, oils	Fatty poultry
Milk, cream, yogurt	Pasta, rice, noodles

Cooking tips: Because this diet is so restrictive, you're going to have to use every trick in the book to make your daily fare as interesting as possible. If you have never had veal, do so now—that is, if you can afford it. If you have never made a roast leg of lamb, now is the time to get out the old recipe book and learn how. I don't mean for all this to sound schoolbookish; it's not. I used the Stillman Diet as an opportunity to find out how to shop for meat. I haunted the meat department at my supermarket every day, made friends with the butcher, an old gentleman only too happy to answer my beginner's questions, and today when anyone says "marbled" to me, my thoughts turn first to steak, and *then* to Italy. So you see, the approach is everything.

Diet hints: One of the side effects of the Stillman Diet is unpleasant mouth odor, which some dieters experience temporarily as a result of intaking only proteins, with no carbohydrates. Though annoying, this condition isn't dangerous. Use a breath spray or breath mint, and rinse frequently with mouthwash. And drink that water—it helps, too.

Also, as on all low-carbohydrate diets, you may experience some constipation, as these are low-roughage diets. Take a stool softener or a very *mild* laxative to correct this situation if it bothers you. But remember, frequent use of laxatives isn't recommended, especially on the Stillman Diet, where dehydrating your system is definitely against policy!

If you feel very weak, take a small glass of orange

juice for instant energy. Though on the "*not* permitted" list, orange juice may be taken in the case of fatigue and/or dizziness.

Let me say again that Dr. Stillman's Quick Weight-loss Diet is one of the very best programs for taking off pounds and inches fast—expect to lose between seven and 15 pounds after the first week, and then five pounds every week after that that you stay on the diet! Should you wish to know more about this diet, you may want to buy *The Doctor's Quick Weight Loss Diet* (Prentice-Hall, hardcover; Dell, paperback).

Dr. Stillman's 14-Day Shape-up Program

If you sneaked and cheated on the Quick Weight-loss Diet, there's good news for you, and it comes in the form of Dr. Stillman's follow-up diet: a 14-day pounds-off program that puts back the foods you missed most on his celebrated Water Diet—vegetables, salad, milk, yogurt, bread and liquor. Latch on to this diet and you can expect to lose between 10 and 25 pounds in two short weeks! Rules are still strict, but the additions to the "permitted" list may finally allow you to succeed in losing weight—cheating won't be necessary.

As an adjunct to his diet, Dr. Stillman, working with co-author Samm Sinclair Baker, devised an exercise program to firm you up as flab is melting away. It's not possible to print these exercises here, but they appear with illustrations and easy how-to directions in Dr. Stillman's book, *Dr. Stillman's 14-Day Shape-Up Program* (Delacorte, hardcover, Dell, paperback).

Following are the diet basics. You don't count either calories or carbohydrates; you eat until you are full at mealtime; you are allowed three meals per day, no snacking in between; and you are permitted to choose *only* from the list of foods below:

Permitted:
Meat: Pure meat, including a variety of meats such as kidneys, sweetbreads and brains. All-beef frankfurters are allowed; luncheon meats, such as salami or bol-

ogna, are not. Cook meats until well done, and trim off visible fat before eating.

Poultry: Only chicken and turkey! No duck, goose or other fatty birds. Cook by broiling, boiling, baking or roasting—you may *not* fry or otherwise use butter or oil. Remove skin before eating.

Fish: Most fish is fine, but you may not have fish packed in oil—sardines, tuna or salmon. In preparing fish, butter may *not* be used.

Seafood: Clams, crabmeat, lobster, mussels, oysters, scallops and shrimp *are* permitted. Although you may not cook these with butter, a small amount of catsup or cocktail sauce is allowed in serving.

Eggs: As long as they are prepared without butter or margarine, eggs may be consumed in unlimited quantities. Those dieters with high cholesterol levels should limit themselves to three eggs per week.

Vegetables: Two cups per day, selected from the following list:

asparagus	Chinese cab-	mushrooms
bamboo shoots	bage	mustard greens
bean sprouts	chives	parsley
beans, wax or	collards	peppers
string	cucumber	radishes
beet greens	eggplant	sauerkraut
broccoli	endive	spinach
brussels sprouts	escarole	summer
cabbage	fennel	squash
cauliflower	kale	tomatoes
celery	kohlrabi	turnip greens
chard	lettuce	watercress
chicory		zucchini

Have one cup of vegetables at lunch, one at dinner. You can choose a half-cup each of two vegetables, instead of one cup of one kind. *No* butter, please, in serving.

Cottage cheese: Any style cottage cheese except the type mixed with fruit or salad greens. Cottage cheese is the only cheese allowed.

Milk: Permitted is one 4 oz. glass of skimmed milk or buttermilk per day. Alternatively, you may have one-half cup of *plain* yogurt. If you like, flavor with artificially sweetened jam.

Bread: Two slices of protein (protogen) bread per day. Dr. Stillman gives his own recipe for Protein-PLUS bread and buns in his book.

Beverages: Water; artificially sweetened soft drinks; bouillon, broth or consommé (3 cups daily); coffee or tea (up to 5 cups daily); milk (see above).

Alcoholic beverages: You may drink 1½ ounces daily of bourbon, brandy, cognac, scotch, rye, Canadian whiskey, Irish whiskey, gin, vodka, tequila or rum (take these liquors straight up). *Or,* instead, a 3 oz. glass of dry white or red wine. You must have one or the other, *not* both.

Desserts: Sugar-free gelatin is the only dessert permitted on the Stillman Shape-up.

Miscellaneous: Sugarless jams and preserves; up to three black or green olives daily; limited amounts of condiments such as catsup, chili sauce, cocktail sauce, mustard, low-calorie salad dressings (no more than a teaspoonful per salad); vinegar; lemon and lime (in moderation); salt, pepper, herbs and sugarless spices.

Anything *not* appearing on the preceding list is out! Oh, yes, Dr. Stillman does make one small concession to candy-lovers—two sticks of sugarless chewing gum per day. Remember, only two, so space them out to make the chews last!

Like the Quick Weight-loss Diet, this plan's fat-less. Butter, margarine, vegetable oils and food items that contain natural oils are strictly prohibited. The difference is that, unlike the QWL, small amounts of carbohydrates *are* allowed. Go by the rules—and take a multivitamin capsule daily (if you're over 40, have a "therapeutic" capsule with lots of B-complex vitamins).

This is a sample menu—be as inventive as you like, mix and match foods to create 14 of your own exciting menus, one for each day of the diet. Some dieters really enjoy sitting down with pencil and paper and working out specific meal plans at the start of a diet. I'm one of these—it gives me a sense of the length of the diet (I can see an end *immediately*), and makes shopping a once-a-week outing.

Sample Menu for the Stillman Shape-up

Breakfast

cottage cheese mixed with sugar-free blueberry preserves
1 slice protogen bread
coffee, tea, skim milk or buttermilk

Lunch

small shrimp cocktail
slice cold poached salmon
cucumber slices, celery stalks, olives
tomato wedges, with vinegar dressing and basil
gelatin dessert
coffee or tea

Dinner

beef consommé with chopped chives
broiled rosemary chicken
spinach and hard-boiled egg salad with dressing
3 oz. Pouilly Fuissé wine (dry white)
coffee or tea

Happy reducing!

Diet hints: Invest in an inexpensive tape measure and gauge the progress of your diet by measuring inches lost. Every three days, check your proportions—especially those areas where bumps and bulges are sorely apparent. If you're not slimming by inches as well as pounds, try some spot-reducing exercises for trouble areas like thighs, stomach, midriff, derrière . . . you can toe-touch or deep knee-bend, but I really don't recommend very strenuous exercise while you're on this diet.

The Mayo Diet

I got a copy of this diet in the mail from a college friend who was living in Boston in 1968—"the hottest diet in my graduate school department," she described it. Well, I was already on the same diet, which was "the hottest diet in my office" that particular week. This one does seem to make the rounds. Nobody's quite sure where it originated, and although it's been called "The Mayo Diet," the famous Minnesota clinic has politely refused credit for this low-gram plan. Wherever it did start, the diet's persisted because of its nearly infallible results: you should lose 10 pounds in as many days, if you keep to these rules. They're easy to follow, and meals are usually put together in just a few short minutes, which is why the diet is a big hit with career people and students.

Breakfast: To start the day, have a half-grapefruit or one cup of unsweetened grapefruit juice. Then two eggs and two slices of bacon (if you're ravenous, have three eggs and three slices of bacon). One cup of coffee or tea.

Lunch: This meal, too, begins with a half-grapefruit. You may have pure meat, cooked any way you like, in unlimited quantities; as much salad as you want with a sugar-free dressing. Coffee or tea.

Dinner: Again, this meal starts with a half-grapefruit. The main course includes any kind of pure meat, poultry or fish, cooked any style. You may have gravy with your meat, if it isn't thickened with flour. Unlimited quantities of red, green or yellow vegetables are permitted and as much salad as you want. Coffee or tea.

Please note that you must *include every item on this menu* for the best possible slimming results; the diet depends on the interaction of these particular types of foods to burn up excess fats in the body. Don't eliminate any food!

Eat until you feel satisfied, until you feel you just couldn't deal with another mouthful. There's no between-meal snacking on the Mayo Diet, so you've got to get it all in at breakfast, lunch and dinner.

You may have butter, margarine or oils on this diet. Meat may be fried, if you wish, and you may add a dab or two of butter to vegetables for flavor. You may also have three tablespoons of heavy cream daily—I'd suggest using it in your coffee or tea, since milk or lemon are not permitted. And on the subject of coffee, the restriction is one cup per meal, and absolutely no more. For can't-do-without-it people, switch to a decaffeinated brand after your third cup of the day. You really must, if you want fat to burn down as quickly as possible.

Permitted: Only the foods which appear on the three menus above, and those listed additionally, such as butter. Anything else is prohibited on this quickie reducing plan.

Cooking tips: On this high-protein plan, meat (or poultry or fish) is the essential item on your lunch and dinner menus. So as not to become dulled to your food, it's a good idea to vary cooking methods as much as you can; don't *always* broil your meat and don't *always* broil your chicken. As I've suggested before for so many of these low-carbo diets, use your diet time to learn how to cook meat, poultry and fish. The knowledge will stand you in good stead for the rest of your life.

Following are some hints and cooking tips I've picked up along the way. Ask friends, older or more experienced cooks, even your mother(!), for their special cooking tricks. Every cook has her bagful and is only too glad to pass along "the best way" to cook anything. Here's my own primer on protein—meats, poultry and fish. Not complete by any means, but you fill in the gaps.

Meat: As I've said before, a good butcher is your best teacher about meat. Befriend yours; ask questions, about value, taste, cooking methods. Believe me, they know *everything!* I began at ground zero, and even had to learn what different grades of meat signified. If you're concerned about protein nutrients, be assured that you can buy any grade of meat and expect the same quality of protein (except that more expensive cuts of meat, with more fat, probably have less protein *per pound*). Protein is protein, and that's that. Grading only means a difference in taste—some cuts are more delicious than others. There are six grades of meat, according to U.S.D.A. standards, but we're really only concerned with the first four:

Prime meat is terribly expensive, but also the most delectable type of meat. If you've never had a prime steak, treat yourself to it once, just for the experience. Prime meat is usually well marbled with fat and encased in a shell of white fat. Of course, as with all grades of meat, it's marked "Prime," as others are marked according to their grade.

Choice is the next desirable cut with less fat than prime and a generally darker color. Choice meat is tender and full of flavor, too.

Good still designates a tasty, tender grade of meat. Leaner than either Prime or Choice, Good grade meat is also darker in color, with a shell of yellow fat.

Standard grade has less flavor than either Choice, Prime, or Good. This grade is hardly marbled at all, and its fat shell is rather skimpy. You should tenderize Standard grades by marinating and seasoning prior to cooking—the longer the better. If you're prepared to put in a bit of work, this grade meat can be made fairly tasty.

Learn your herbs and seasonings. As embellishments to meat, they're marvelous when properly used. One of my own best tricks is to cut a clove of garlic into thin slivers, then wedge these slivers into deep cuts I've made in steaks or roasts. Push the garlic into each cut with a knife so the sliver is invisible. Cook the meat as usual; the garlic, permeating the surrounding flesh, adds a wonderful delicate taste.

Poultry: Best to buy fresh poultry—it's much tastier than packaged birds. If you're buying at the supermarket, though, prefer poultry with a federal inspection stamp; though law doesn't require stamping, their presence indicates certain adherence to grading standards. Again, ask the "meat man" (every low-carbo dieter's best friend) if you have further questions.

Birds (chickens, that is) are classified by weight. The sex and age of the bird also determine whether it is called a broiler, fryer, roaster or capon. *Broilers* and *fryers* are young chickens, male or female. Broilers weigh up to 2½ pounds; fryers are between 2½ and 3½ pounds. *Roasters* are larger, between 3½ and 5 pounds; and *capons* are castrated male birds weighing between 6 and 8 pounds. Capons are plump and fully-fleshed. Check any good cookbook for specific ways to cook poultry. I still find Rombauer's *Joy of Cooking* incredibly useful in explaining cooking basics.

Fish: You can buy fish whole, halved, filleted or cut into steaks. If you live by the water, you're lucky to be guaranteed fresh fish daily; for inland-dwellers, your best bet is a fish market (rather than a supermarket), where fish is undoubtedly as fresh as it can be. Consult the "fish man" (or woman, now that I think about it!) if you have any questions about how much to buy, how to cook and so on. Here are some cooking tips which you may not know.

1. When you broil fish, such as halibut or salmon steak, use a high, intense heat rather than a low fire. Quick cooking retains the flavor of the fish, and it tastes better.

2. Steaming and poaching are fine methods for delicate fish. These methods cook by moist heat; the difference is that in poaching, the fish is immersed in the near-boiling liquid, while in steaming it is not.

3. Test your fish with a thermometer to see if it is cooked. Between 140–145°F signifies doneness—cooked longer, flavor and juices escape. Or use a toothpick to test: insert in the thickest part of the meat; if flesh flakes and appears to be solid in color, the fish is ready.

4. To cut a very fishy taste, use lemon, vinegar, and garlic. Marinate fish and/or season in cooking.

The Seven-day Chicken Diet

There are a lot of chicken jokes around these days, but this diet is definitely not one of them! This low-carb plan knows more ways to fix a chicken than you have excuses for *not* losing weight. Go with this super-cheap, super-easy reducing plan and you can expect to lose at least five pounds per week. You eat chicken every day of the week, and also rely on grapefruit, eggs and salad to whisk pounds away. Other menu items are gram-low, too, and supremely easy to prepare. If you're the lone dieter in your family, you can serve these menus to the whole gang, adding other foods such as rice and potatoes and desserts for the non-dieters.

Following is a week's worth of menus. Designed to

minimize cooking time, you can prepare chicken for two or three days' worth of menus all at the same time. For example, roast a chicken on Monday, eat it cold in chicken salad sandwich on Tuesday, and heat it on Wednesday for chow mein!

Monday

Breakfast
1 poached egg on
1 slice toast
2 bacon strips
coffee or tea

Lunch
1 broiled hamburger
tomato wedges
tossed green salad
coffee or tea

Dinner
½ grapefruit
6 oz. roast chicken
endive salad
4 oz. dry white wine

Tuesday

Breakfast
1 cup cottage cheese
  with sugar-free
  strawberry preserves
coffee or tea

Lunch
½ grapefruit
cucumber salad
chicken salad sandwich
coffee or tea

Dinner
4 oz. minute steak
1 cup spinach
1 cup cauliflower
4 oz. dry red wine

Wednesday

Breakfast
1 slice French toast
  with sugar-free jelly
  or jam
coffee or tea

Lunch
small shrimp cocktail
large spinach, bacon, hard-
  boiled egg salad
coffee or tea

Dinner
1 cup chicken chow mein
  with ¼ cup rice
¼ cantaloupe with lemon
  wedge
coffee or tea

Thursday

Breakfast
½ grapefruit
2 scrambled eggs
2 bacon strips
coffee or tea

Lunch
1 broiled chicken breast
2 broiled tomato halves
tossed salad
4 oz. dry white wine

Dinner
1 cheeseburger on bun
endive salad
coffee or tea

Friday

Breakfast
1 cup cottage cheese
1 slice toast
coffee or tea

Lunch
½ grapefruit
2 lamb chops
1 cup broccoli
coffee or tea

Dinner
1 cup chicken à la king
1 slice toast
coffee or tea

Saturday

Breakfast
1 poached egg on
1 slice toast topped
  with hot, stewed
  tomatoes
coffee or tea

Lunch
½ cantaloupe with
1 scoop cottage cheese
coffee or tea

Dinner
6 oz. roast chicken
1 cup broccoli
escarole salad
4 oz. dry red wine

Sunday

Breakfast
jelly omelette (made
  with 2 eggs, sugar-
  free jelly)
coffee or tea

Lunch
4 oz. any type steak
  with wine and mushroom
  sauce
½ cup spinach
½ cup cauliflower
4 oz. dry red wine

Dinner
1 chicken, tomato and cucumber
  sandwich
coffee or tea

Some more rules . . . you may also have:

1. 2 pats of butter per day.
2. 1 cup skim milk per day.
3. 3 cups coffee per day—no more than that!
4. 1 slice lemon or lime daily.
5. Unlimited quantities of water, broth or bouillon and sugar-free carbonated beverages.
6. Seasonings and condiments: all herbs and sugar-free spices. Catsup, barbecue sauce, cocktail sauce, Worcestershire sauce, all in moderation.

The Great Hamburger Diet

Is there anyone who doesn't love a hamburger? Every one of my friends who's tried this low-gram plan comes back applauding it—with skinnier cheers and claps. It's the simplest low-carb diet of them all: stick to the menu given for seven days, and watch the scales slide down a whopping five pounds or more. Some folks may find repeating the same breakfasts, lunches and dinners far too dull, but personally, I find the Hamburger Diet's sameness and predictability reassuring. And if you adore burgers as I do and know a few gourmet tricks to add flavor interest, there couldn't be a more delightful way to slim (I'll give you my own tips later).

As with all diets, you should have your doctor's OK before embarking on the Great Hamburger Diet. Do take a multivitamin capsule each day of your diet, eat only the meals listed below and drink water by the glassfuls to help wash away that flab.

THE GREAT HAMBURGER DIET MENUS

Breakfast	Lunch
½ grapefruit	1 large all-beef hamburger
1 cup cottage cheese	lettuce and tomato salad
2 slices unsalted melba toast	1 cup skim milk
black coffee or tea	

Dinner
1 large all-beef hamburger
2 vegetables (from list below)
black coffee or tea

Select two vegetables from among these—you may have one cup of each vegetable for dinner:

asparagus	kale
beans, string or wax	lettuce
bean sprouts	mushrooms
beet greens	mustard greens
broccoli	okra
cabbage	peppers, green
cauliflower	spinach
celery	squash, summer
chard	turnip greens
cucumber	water chestnuts
eggplant	watercress

When shopping for your hamburger meat, buy either ground round or ground sirloin, perhaps a bit more expensive than chuck, but the reduced fat content will speed your diet along at the proper rate. Give zest to burgers by adding herbs and seasonings before you cook: pepper, garlic powder or minced garlic clove, onion flakes, Worcestershire or A-1 sauce or chili sauce should be mixed together with the raw ground beef. Then cook your burger under a hot broiler flame, or pan-fry—no butter or oil, just a few shakes of salt in your pan will draw out enough natural fat for cooking. You are allowed one tablespoon of catsup, barbecue sauce, mustard or chili sauce with each hamburger. Pickles, relishes and other condiments are *not* permitted.

Permitted: Only those items listed on the Hamburger Diet menus *plus:* unlimited quantities of water, club soda, sugar-free carbonated beverages, broth or bouillon *and* one teaspoon of your favorite salad dressing for noon-time salad.

Not permitted: Foods not included in the listings above. No butter, margarine, or oils. No bread (except for breakfast melba toast). No fruits (beside a half-grapefruit). No substitute meat. No sweets. No alcohol, and so on. I'm sure you know which foods you'll have to forego for this week.

Diet hints: This is another super diet for working people. Hamburgers are available in most every coffee shop I know, as are simple salads—and that effort-saving burger dinner is a boon when all you want to do is collapse after that proverbial "hard day at the office."

THE OUT-AND-OUT CRASH DIETS

Crashing is the only way some people can do it. If you've toyed with the idea of dieting, but never actually got around to the diet itself, a crash may be the shove your lazy soul needs. Or if a bonus five pounds is keeping you zipped *out* of the good dress you must wear to your cousin's wedding next weekend, relax. An out-and-out crash diet will reduce you fast. These are the emergency measures that have gotten thousands of us out of the same "tight" spot.

Only one week on a crash, remember—and you should be in sparkling good health. See your doctor for his seal of approval. Talk to him if you want to stay on a crash for more than a week.

As well as being practically fool-proof, crash diets will keep you far removed from temptation. You can shop just once and pick up everything the diet requires, and from then on your only decisions will be: should I slice this banana or eat it whole? Should I fry my egg this morning or poach it? Some people call these idiot diets, and you can see why. If you're not the world's greatest decision-maker, a crash program may be the surest way for you to reduce.

In choosing a crash diet, consider your taste buds. Since you'll be eating exactly the same foods every day, make sure your stomach agrees with your selection. If you loathe cottage cheese, for example, it doesn't make much sense to pick the Cottage Cheese Blitz. Crashing shouldn't be punishment, but should offer you the foods you genuinely enjoy.

No matter which crash you decide on, take a multiple-vitamin-mineral pill once a day, or twice a day if you're over 40. Drink lots of water and other calorie-free liquids. Give up liquor (unless you choose the Egg and Wine Diet). Eliminate salt from your diet, or use a salt-substitute. Go to bed early—and I mean that, too; if you're asleep you won't know you're hungry, and besides, you need lots of energy for these ultra-low calorie plans.

A final word: if you have a few more days to lose that extra weight, adjust the diet accordingly, adding small quantities of the *same* foods to each meal. Otherwise, these diets are three-day to one-week plans, as indicated. One week to a slim, trim figure.

The Meat and Mushroom Diet

Mad for meat? Maniacal about mushrooms? Then this two-dish crash may be *your* dish. The MMD debuted in *Look* (March 1962), and for a decade its fans have used it to trim five pounds in five days. Here's how the plan works. You are permitted only the following foods:

Meat: You may have up to nine ounces of meat a day—100% pure beef, lamb or veal, trimmed of all fat. Very lean bacon and Canadian bacon are fine, too, but limit these to two ounces of either daily. Cook the meat without butter or oil—broiling, boiling, roasting, baking or frying in a Teflon pan are all good methods. For best results, distribute your nine-ounce quota evenly: have three ounces of meat for breakfast, three ounces for lunch, etc.

Mushrooms: If you're using fresh mushrooms, you may have 18–24 medium-sized ones per day. The limit for canned varieties is one and a half cups, drained of all liquid. Bake or broil mushrooms—again, no fat or butter allowed—or enjoy them *au naturel*—raw!

Permitted: To perk up meat and mushrooms, you may add one half-cup per day of chopped onions, green peppers, spinach, tomatoes, asparagus or green beans. And you may have one tablespoon of either sour cream, plain yogurt or grated Parmesan cheese. Seasonings such as lemon juice, herbs and spices are permitted, too, but no salt. Instant bouillon or broth is fine between meals and/or before you retire.

The Skim Milk and Banana Diet

This out-and-out crash dates back a minimum of 30 years (I know because I can remember my grandmother going on it), but despite its fame and longevity, I haven't been able to track down where or when the diet started, or who deserves credit for it. All I can tell you for sure is that this is one of the crash classics: a simple, bland-food plan on which you can shed up to five pounds in just three days. Here's how you do it.

Bananas: Four bananas per day are allowed—average-sized. For best results, have a banana morning, noon, evening and mid-evening; schedule your milk for in-between hours.

Skim milk: Three eight-ounce glasses a day. Remember, you can't have whole milk, only skim. If the taste isn't one you like, add a teaspoon of coffee flavoring, cherry extract, etc.

For a special treat, you may mix one banana and one eight-ounce glass of milk in your blender to produce a thick, creamy banana shake. I like to start the day with one of these because it seems terribly festive on such a strict regimen!

The Egg and Wine Diet

In 1964, *Vogue* reported this crash to be one of the "seven most-talked about diets of the moment." Years

later, the plan is still making the rounds. By far the
most offbeat of the out-and-out crashes, the Egg and
Wine doesn't have mass appeal, but if you're overweight
and a wine connoisseur, too, you may enjoy trying it
over a long weekend. The regime is super-slimming
and, to quote one of my more fashionable friends, "positively *smashing,* my dear!"

First thing in the morning, uncork a small (24-
ounce) bottle of dry wine—white, red or rosé. Sip a
cup of black coffee or tea while you soft-cook or poach
an egg. Eat your egg; toast yourself ("To my slimness!") with a six-ounce glass of wine. Repeat the same
procedure at noon, but have two eggs instead of one; at
dinner, it's two eggs again—or, if you just can't—a tiny
steak. As for the wine, finish the bottle. And sleep well.

If it's too much wine for you, or if you want an even
quicker-working crash, spread that bottle of wine over
two days, instead of one.

The Cottage Cheese Blitz

Anyone who's ever dieted knows about cottage
cheese. It's undoubtedly the country's #1 diet food.
And of all the many cottage cheese diets—you'd be
amazed at how many there are—the Blitz is probably
the best known and most successful. From the book by
Ruth West, *Stop Dieting! Start Losing!* (Dutton, hardcover; Bantam, paperback), this crash plan promises
no-nonsense results. Even if you're not that crazy about
cottage cheese, look at it this way: you can lose as
much as five pounds in two days. Couldn't you learn to
love it just a little?

This is maximum crash dieting. Breakfast, lunch and
dinner puts this same meal on your plate:

    ¾ cup skim-milk cottage cheese
    1 portion fruit or vegetable
    2 crackers

A portion of fresh fruit includes one of the following:
a small tangerine or pineapple slice; two apricots or

dried prunes; a half-cup fresh berries; half a small cantaloupe, grapefruit or orange (or a half-cup of sections). Substitute canned fruit if you find it easier—a half-cup of anything water-packed or artificially sweetened.

A portion of vegetables means as big a serving as you want of radishes, green peppers, cucumbers, scallions, celery and lettuce. Many dieters enjoy dicing a mix of these very fine and combining them with cottage cheese. Also permissible: a medium-sized tomato or a large carrot.

Limit your choice of crackers to saltines, melba toast, rye or wheat thins. If it makes you happy, top them with dietetic jelly.

Enhance the flavor of plain cottage cheese with a sprinkle of nutmeg or cinnamon to satisfy your nagging sweet tooth; chives, fresh pepper and assorted herbs create a spicy taste.

The Steak and Tomato Diet

Of all the "Steak and . . ." diets around, I believe this plan offers the most variety. Credit for this delightful duo goes to the old *Liberty* magazine, circa 1944 (or was it the *Saturday Evening Post*?). Well, whoever invented it, this shed-a-pound-a-day plan works. Here's how.

Steak: London broil for lunch? Sirloin for supper? It's up to you—just so long as the meat is 100% lean beef and you trim off all visible fat. No matter what preparation method you use, do it without oil, fat or butter, and discard all pan drippings.

You are permitted nine ounces of steak daily, or eight ounces for a faster-working diet. The diet originally called for a whopping 12 ounces of steak, but in the 1940s a woman of five feet four inches was considered svelte at 130 pounds. If times and the numbers have changed, be assured that steak hasn't. It's still one of the best diet foods around.

Tomatoes: Four medium-size tomatoes are your daily ration. Be experimental. Stew them, braise them, bake them, broil them. Eat them raw if you prefer, or

drink them (you can substitute a six-ounce glass of tomato juice for each tomato).

Seasonings: Go ahead and season your steak and tomatoes with herbs, spices and lemon juice. The tomatoes can be braised in bouillon or stewed with green
pepper. If you wish, enjoy your steak with a few fresh
or broiled onion slices; dip it in a teaspoon or two—no
more—of mustard, catsup or Worcestershire or meat
sauce.

Etc. Have a salad with your steak: carve up tomatoes,
add cucumbers, scallions and lettuce; sprinkle with vinegar, lemon juice or a low-calorie dressing.

You are also permitted one cup of vegetable each
day, prepared by steaming, boiling or baking. Choose
from among these: asparagus, broccoli spears, spinach
or zucchini.

The Egg and Orange Diet

Back in the early 1950s, this full-scale crash was very
popular with sun-worshippers along the exclusive
French Riviera resorts. Later the plan appeared in *Elle*
(a chic French magazine) as one of three "beautiful
people" diets and, sometime in the late 1950s, this established European classic finally reached dieters on the
far side of the Atlantic.

Stick to the Egg and Orange Diet faithfully and you
should drop five pounds in a mere three days. Here are
your daily menus. No substitutions are permitted.

Breakfast	*Lunch*
½ cup orange sections	1 cup instant bouillon
6 oz. glass skim milk	1 egg
	1 orange or 2 tangerines

Dinner
6 oz. tomato juice
2 eggs
½ head lettuce; ½ cucumber
1 orange or 2 tangerines

Eggs may be cooked any style, so long as you don't
use butter, margarine or fat in their preparation.

The Gourmet Diet

If you're rich, this crash plan will delight you. When money is no object, the Gourmet Diet will let you eat like royalty and shrink by as many as five pounds in three days. The idea for the Gourmet Crash stems from *Esquire* (June 1963); however, the original plan was designed to last seven days and trimmed only three or four pounds. This modified version works faster and is a bit less expensive than the original.

Breakfast
½ grapefruit topped with cinnamon
2 oz. smoked salmon slices

Lunch
4 oz. glass of (*brut*) champagne
2 tbsp. red or black caviar on
2 slices of melba toast
demitasse oolong tea

Dinner
4 oz. glass of (*brut*) champagne
1 tbsp. paté atop
2 melba rounds
4 oz. broiled shrimp, lobster or crab with lemon-garlic sauce
½ cup fresh blueberries with
1 tbsp. whipped cream
espresso

The Strawberry and Cream Diet

According to hearsay, this summertime crash plan made its first appearance in the now defunct *Woman's Home Companion*. The diet, however, is still very much alive, and I can swear that it works, and works fast. Here is the version I follow when I need to shrink down quickly for Labor Day weekend.

Your daily allotment of strawberries is five cups. You may not sweeten fruit, except with artificial sweeteners. If fresh berries are not available where you live, frozen strawberries may be substituted only if they have been left whole without syrup or sugar added.

Most traditionalists use sour cream on this diet; however, you may use light sweet cream if you prefer, or switch back and forth as you wish. Plain yogurt is perfectly fine, too, as is whipped cream. Whichever you decide on, your allowance is up to (but not more than) eight tablespoons every day.

I recommend having one cup of berries and cream for breakfast; a second cup at noon; and two cups at dinner. This schedule will give you an extra cup to divide up as between-meal snacks or for nibbling.

This crash plan is a three-day quickie. If you're faithful, you can expect to be five pounds trimmer at the end of that time.

Diet hint: Make it a point to use sour cream or yogurt on the diet. If you do, you can eke out a midmorning snack. Have your breakfast berries without any topping; later on enjoy the yogurt or sour cream you've saved with chopped scallions or radishes.

The Yogurt Diet

Deliciously cool and creamy yogurt is one of the world's most superb diet foods. Follow this tasty yogurt crash, and you can expect to see the scales fall five pounds over one long 3-day weekend! While slimming you down, yogurt also does other good, healthy things for the body—it provides the dieter with a bounty of protein, calcium and vitamin A, and also serves to cleanse the digestive tract. Remember, you are allowed only the three items listed below. No more, less if you like—but no substitutions.

Each day you may have four cups of plain yogurt. Fruit or fruit-flavored yogurts are not permitted, since they contain up to twice the number of calories as unflavored plain.

In addition, you may have one whole medium cantaloupe.

Eat these foods separately, or combine them at mealtime. You might choose to organize your menus like this, for instance:

> *Breakfast:* ¼ cantaloupe, sliced, and topped with 1 cup yogurt
> *Mid-morning:* ½ cup yogurt with artificial sweetener
> *Lunch:* ¼ cantaloupe, sliced, topped with 1 cup yogurt
> *Dinner:* ½ cantaloupe with 1 cup yogurt
> *Late-evening:* ½ cup yogurt with artificial sweetener

Like the Strawberry and Cream Crash, the Yogurt Diet is an ideal plan for summer months, when cantaloupe—fresh and sweet—is widely available and relatively inexpensive.

The Ice Cream Diet

I told you there was a pounds-off plan for ice cream lovers and here it is! If you can't give ice cream up for anything, go with your passion and lose 10 pounds in one short week. The ice cream crash works this way:

Every day, you are allowed to eat three cups of ice cream, any flavor you choose. (French ice cream which is higher in fat content is not your best friend.)

One way to stretch your ice cream allowance is to enjoy six mini-meals a day; ½ cup of ice cream per meal. Stock your freezer with all your favorite flavors—vanilla fudge, butter pecan, pistachio, peppermint swirl . . . Making that delectable choice six times each day will keep you from getting bored with this crash, one of the lushest ways to lose weight!

As with all crash plans, consult your doctor first. If you have to limit saturated fats because of cholesterol levels, this out-and-out crash isn't for you—you'd do better with one of the other fast-working plans in this section.

The Hamburger Crash Diet

Similar to the low-carbohydrate Hamburger Diet (page 117), the Hamburger Crash cuts out the frills to enable you to lose weight even quicker. Nothing is permitted on this diet except hamburger. You may have three large hamburgers each day, and nothing else! One for breakfast, a second at lunchtime and a third whopping burger for dinner. Season your burgers with salt, pepper, herbs, spices and Worcestershire or A-1 sauce, and prepare by broiling or frying (without butter or fat) in a Teflon pan.

You should drink lots of water on this out-and-out crash and you may have unlimited glassfuls of artifically sweetened carbonated beverages.

This diet has been used with fabulous success in a famous Boston obesity clinic—pounds disappear overnight, while you hardly experience any hunger at all. Protein—which hamburger is—takes longer to digest than other food nutrients, making the time between meals seem very short indeed. I go on this crash periodically, as do many of my friends—and I swear to you, it works!

THE NO-PLAN DIET: FASTING

To take off weight really fast, fast! Abstaining from food is one great way to switch yourself into "diet psych," the slim frame of mind that many dieters claim is the key to reducing success. With an initial surge of weight loss, fasting provides such a radical change, such a total break from past habits of overindulgence, that many overweights find it the ideal way to get a diet really rolling. You won't collapse from hunger, nor will you faint in the street, but after eight hours without a solid bite to eat, you will, if you're like most people, experience a marvelous sense of well-being and calm. And excess pounds will just be falling away.

Consult your doctor first. If you are ill or run down,

you shouldn't fast. But if your doctor approves, join the ranks of famous fasters like Mae West, Van Johnson and Edie Adams who abstain regularly—either to take off weight or to maintain a slim figure. Should your physician wish to supervise your fast, follow his instructions. Otherwise, tell him about the at-home fast I describe here, and see if he approves of it for you. If he does, you'll need to follow these simple rules.

1. Take a high-potency multiple vitamin each day.

2. Avoid strenuous physical and/or mental activity. Walking is permitted, even recommended, but high-pitch exercise like jogging or tennis should be put off. I like to fast over the weekend when pressures from the job and other commitments can be happily locked away.

3. Get lots of sleep. Though you will probably feel a surge of energy after about six or seven hours without food, don't push your body. Eight hours of sleep is a requirement.

4. Drink plenty of water, tea, club soda and other calorie-free beverages.

5. Get lots of fresh air. Purify your lungs, too, with clean, country air—if you can! Many people prefer fasting during the spring and summer months when they can spend long hours outdoors.

If you're eating nothing at all and drinking only water, don't fast for longer than 24 hours. Staying on a water fast for days or weeks is advisable only within a closely supervised hospital situation, where your progress may be closely monitored. Fast for one day—drinking pure mountain spring water—to inaugurate your regular diet program. You'll lose a pound or several pounds, "shrink" your stomach a bit and be absolutely rarin' to succeed on your own diet. There are no real rules for fasting, except those I've just mentioned. You don't eat anything—not a bit of food—and drink as much water and as many calorie-free beverages as you care to have. Expect to feel hungry for the first few hours of your fast; dizziness, lightheadedness and headache are common complaints during this initial period. Happily, these symptoms disappear after several hours, and you're left with an unmistakable sense of calm, and no desire to eat.

Fasting with water is certainly effective, but I prefer this traditional European juice fast, which allows me to enjoy aromatic herbal teas and fresh juices as well as water. Juice fasts are easier on the system—they're calorie-*low,* not calorie-less, as the fruit and vegetable juices permitted contain food energy as well as nutrients. So, while you're not actually eating in the sense of biting and chewing, you are taking in nourishment. You won't lose quite so much weight as with a water fast, but you will lose and still *feel* you're not eating at all— one of the great psychological benefits of fasting.

Start the day with a piping hot cup of herbal tea. Health food stores, even supermarkets nowadays, carry a wondrous variety of herb teas which you can prepare exactly as you would regular tea. If you can't buy tea bags, loose tea may be steeped in a teapot or infused in a cup of hot water with a "tea ball." Camomile, peppermint, rose hips and alfalfa are the herbal teas most people like, although other more esoteric types are fun to try out, too.

At mid-morning, have an eight-ounce glass of fresh fruit juice. Freshly-squeezed orange or grapefruit juice, costlier than canned or frozen, is well worth the added pennies. Since this is all you'll be having, why not treat yourself like royalty?

For lunch, a bowl of chicken or beef broth or consommé, or, if you like, an eight-ounce glass of vegetable juice. Tomato, V-8, carrot, carrot mixed with apple, even sauerkraut juices are fine; you're lucky if you own a juice extractor, which allows you to make your own fresh vegetable juices. If not, canned juices are delicious when chilled.

Mid-afternoon, have another cup of herbal tea, and for dinner, choose between a tall glass of fruit or vegetable juice. Before going to bed, I usually sip some camomile tea, one of nature's own best tranquilizers.

Fast for two or three days, and that's all. Controlled fasting is safe, but you must be watched by a doctor if you wish to continue for longer than three days.

When you are ready to break your fast, don't eat anything too heavy. Bland, soft foods like scrambled eggs, cooked cereal, spaghetti or noodles or a piece of fruit are recommended as a first meal. Ease yourself back into normal foods, a little at a time. Remember, your stomach has been on vacation; don't shock it with a super-heavy workload.

GROUP-ACTION PLANS

My friend Maggie was a diet disaster area for years. For as long as I'd known her, this gal had been on a diet—or, I should say, *diets,* one after another after another. Each time she "discovered" a new program, it was heralded as the Diet of Diets, the one plan that was finally going to chisel her size 14 figure down to normal proportions. Over the years, I'd listened to glowing recommendations for all kinds of weight-loss schemes, and I'd also seen dozens of diets fall by the wayside. Undaunted, Maggie simply moved on. If amazed, I did admire her boundless optimism because in the same situation, I would have long ago given up altogether.

About a year ago she called me, wildly ecstatic, and enthusiastic in a completely different way. She had lost 15 pounds and was down to a size 10 dress! "You know," she said, "I finally came to the conclusion after 23 diets in five years, that it was me and not the diets. I just couldn't do it alone." How Maggie *did* do it was with Weight Watchers, perhaps the most famous of all the group-action diet plans. She admitted that she needed a group of sympathetic people pushing her to lose weight. "They were all so interested in my problem," she said, "because they were all as fat as me! I knew that they were all behind me, cheering me on, and it made me stick to the diet."

Group-action plans are the easiest way for some of us to lose weight, and if you recognize something of yourself in Maggie, they may be the only way. If you've failed at diets before and can't seem to find a single plan that works for you; if you thrive in social situations; if you believe wholeheartedly that "misery loves company"; if you need encouragement, support and peer approval that you don't get from family and friends—consider dieting in company. There are several nationally known group action plans which hold meetings in most large cities and towns. Even if you're not near to any of these, you can form your own neighborhood diet club with *simpático* friends who also want to slim down.

Shop around. You can usually attend complimentary meetings of any diet group just to try it out. Since groups vary in philosophy and differ in method and ambience, sampling a few groups before commiting yourself to one is a good idea. Weight Watchers, TOPS, The Diet Workshop and Overeaters Anonymous are large organizations with national memberships, and you might want to consider one of these. You can write to them at the addresses listed below for complete information on their programs, but meanwhile—for openers—a brief rundown on each group:

Weight Watchers is the brilliant invention of former housewife Jean Nidetch, now perhaps the world's most famous ex-fattie. A commercial enterprise with franchises all over the world, Weight Watchers has reached over five million overweight people with a technique that has proven wonderfully effective for the faithful and the persistent. Members pay a fee to attend regular weekly meetings (you're fined for meetings missed as incentive to come) where they weigh in, listen to lectures by successful losers, question the diet experts and socialize with other WW reducers. Mutual encouragement, support and understanding, say WW numerous fans, are what make the program tick. As Maggie described it, "Those people respect fat! Or, rather, how serious the problem is. They know; they've been there, too." The WW Diet is a strict 1200-calorie regimen. By following the rules, eating your meat, fish, fruit, veggies, salads and skim milk, you can expect to lose about two and a half pounds each week. For further information, contact Weight Watchers International Inc., 800 Community Drive, Manhasset, New York 11030 (telephone 516–627–9200).

TOPS (Take Off Pounds Sensibly) is a non-profit weight-loss program, and the oldest one in this country. More down to basics than Weight Watchers, TOPS members pay a small annual dues fee and can attend

unlimited meetings, as they wish. Meeting styles very
from chapter to chapter, sometimes including a lecture
by a visiting nutritionist, at other times incorporating
sing-along fests, games and contests. Members weigh in
at each meeting—TOPS emphasizes competition to
lose; prizes are awarded and "titles" conferred on the
individual who's lost the most for a particular week.
TOPS contributes large sums of money for obesity research, news of which members receive in a monthly
newsletter. Otherwise, there is no specific TOPS diet;
individual diets must be supervised by your own doctor.
Buoyed by their medical affiliations, TOPS has also
proved successful in helping members to lose weight.
Write for additional information to TOPS, 4575 S. 5th
St., P.O. Box 4489, Milwaukee, Wisconsin 53207 (telephone 414–482–4620).

The Diet Workshop is more therapy-oriented than
other diet groups. Founders Lois Lyons Lindauer and
Edith Berman feel that as well as providing a workable
diet and peer support, another of Diet Workshop's important functions is to help overweights understand that
compulsive eating patterns *can* and *must* be changed.
They show members how to do this in small group ses-
sions where individual problems are talked out and
suggestions for change discussed. Diet Workshop, with
groups in 25 states, charges a fee for each meeting you
attend, with bargain-rate contracts available on a 10-
week basis. The DW Diet is a well-balanced, low-
calorie regimen with provisions for inveterate snackers,
and there is a special program offered for those who
need to lose just 10 pounds. Write to the Diet Workshop, Inc., 1975 Hempstead Turnpike, East Meadow,
New York 11554 (telephone 516–794–4881).

Overeaters Anonymous is, in theory, a departure
from the three groups described above. The basis for
this nationwide program are other "Anonymous" organizations—Alcoholics Anonymous and Gamblers Anonymous, the direct inspiration for OA's creation. "Taking
one day at a time" is the urgent message; each successful dieting day is a landmark for the OA members.
Meetings, which are free, unless you choose to make a
donation, happen on a regular basis. Members are en-

couraged to talk about their weight problems, diet successes and flops. Like AA and GA, OA encourages belief in a higher spiritual power to help members overcome problems, though belief in a god is certainly no prerequisite for joining OA. There is no one specific OA diet, though a choice of three diets is available to the dieter not under doctor's care. For further information, write to Overeaters Anonymous, 3730 Motor Avenue, Los Angeles, California 90034 (telephone 213–559–6140).

Forming your own diet group may be smarter if you're not within the proximity of an established program or if you prefer rules tailored to your individual needs. One very successful group I know of was started by a woman who worked for a large New York insurance company. Having decided against spending extra money on an organized program, she formed an office diet club and had no trouble soliciting members. Anyone could join so long as she was serious about losing weight, no matter how many or how few pounds needed to be lost. Members selected their own diets and met every Monday and Thursday at lunchtime to discuss their progress. At these get-togethers, members' weights were recorded in a notebook, "cheating" confessed to and discussed and special problems talked over. The only group stipulation was that any advice given to one member by another be positive in nature. By the end of two months, only two of the original 13 members had dropped out, and the remaining 11 had either arrived at their weight goal or were solidly on their way to it. As one of the group members reported, "Dieting with co-workers was great. It saved me and lots of other women from fattening lunches (members ate home-packed diet lunches at meetings), provided on-the-spot encouragement when many of us had no time for other diet groups like Weight Watchers and one of the unexpected bonuses was that we started to work together better than ever before!"

Diet with friends at work, or organize a group in your neighborhood if you're at home during the day. Taking off pounds in good company is the way some (former) overweights have been able to lose accumulated fat forever.

CORINNE'S DIET PLANS

Make up your own diets? Why not! I've been doing it for years, sometimes because I get bored with by-the-book rules, sometimes because I can't find a single diet that suited my tastes and needs of the moment. I remember one college summer, when I was very involved in European-style picnicking: breads, cheeses, wines, fruits, the whole picture. Now while this is a terribly romantic way to dine (your gourmet goodies spread out on a checkered cloth under sunny June skies, sharing subtle taste experiences with a compatible friend), it's also, as they say, *très* fattening. I gained seven pounds that summer and while I realized by August it was time to take that fat off, I wasn't quite prepared to give up my sophisticated picnics—well, you know how it is when you're 18. So, I compromised by inventing the Muenster Cheese and Apple Diet, a picnic diet plan that kept up the spirit of the meal, but sliced calories back to a sensible quota. It's possible to adapt your own food preferences in creating diets. Literally any food can be a diet food if you keep within certain easy rules: Diets must be either low-calorie or low-carbohydrate in nature. If you're making up a low-calorie plan, restrict calories to under 1000 per day. In creating low-carbo diets, keep carbohydrate grams to under 60 per day. It works, believe me!

Following are some of my own creations. If they appeal to you, I'm pleased. If not, use Corinne's Diet Plans to fire your own imagination. As with any diet, check with your doctor first and remember to take a multivitamin pill every day you're dieting.

The Muenster Cheese and Apple Diet

I've explained the origins of this one—it's a marvelous picnic-style plan that works especially well during the summer, or in April and May when you're svelting down for bikini weather. All three meals, breakfast, lunch and dinner, are exactly the same, but you can add interest with different summer-cooler beverages. Iced tea with peppermint, iced coffee whirled in the blender with crushed ice, diet soda with a squeeze of fresh lemon, club soda with a few drops of artificial flavoring or just plain bottled spring water are drinks I've enjoyed with these mini-meals. Stick with this diet for three days and you'll see the scales slide down five whole pounds.

Each diet meal consists of one ounce of muenster cheese and one medium apple. Serve the apple chilled, of course, and make the meal last longer by slicing the fruit into eight or 10 thin wedges and cutting the cheese into bite-size pieces. When I'm feeling really ambitious, I toothpick each and every little cheese chunk.

I recommended this plan to one good friend who improvised on it by slicing the top off the apple, coring it as you would if you were baking it, filling the center with the muenster cheese and sticking the whole thing under the broiler until the apple was tender and the cheese melted within its shell. I can't vouch for this recipe myself, but I also can't see why it wouldn't be delicious.

The French Toast and Banana Blast

This diet harks back, I'm sure, to childhood when mashed bananas were a comforting staple and French toast a favorite breakfast order with my sister Fran and me. Breakfast and dinner on this diet are identical, but you're permitted something different at lunch.

Morning and evening meals consists of a crispy hot slice of French toast topped with mashed banana. Prepare this way: Mash one-half of a medium-sized banana and set aside. Now dip one slice of white bread (a thin slice!) in one egg, beaten. When the bread is soaked, but not crumbling, transfer it to a small frying pan in which you've melted one teaspoon of butter. Fry the toast until golden brown. As it's cooking, spoon the mashed banana into the same pan and fry until it's good and hot. To serve, simply spread the banana over the French toast.

For lunch, I have one cup of fresh fruit cocktail and two slices of unsalted melba toast. Canned fruit cocktail is OK, too, but fresh is infinitely better and more delicious. But, of course, that's up to you.

Black coffee and plain tea are permitted on this diet, as are the standard no- or low-calorie beverages.

Cooking tip: Save the beaten egg, which you won't have used up at breakfast, for making your dinner-time French toast. It's just a few pennies saved, but they add up.

The Thick Shake Shape-up

Malteds and thick shakes let you pretend you're not dieting, because as they're normally prepared—with ice cream, thick chocolate and rich sugary syrups—they're incredibly fattening. This diet preserves the illusion of "fattening" without the calories. You feel like you're getting away with something, and all the while you'll be melting inches off your waistline.

The menu is three shakes a day—follow the recipes I've made up here. The only substitution you can make is to repeat your lunch and dinner shakes. In other words, you can have the banana or the strawberry shake twice in one day, but you may have only one orange shake, which is slightly more fattening.

Breakfast: Prepare your *orange shake* by mixing together in a blender one cup of orange juice, one raw egg, three tablespoons half-and-half and some crushed ice. Blend for one minute. Drink immediately.

Lunch: Your mid-day *banana shake* is made by blending one cup skim milk, one-half of a medium banana and one-half teaspoon vanilla together for one minute. Serve on the spot.

Dinner: Finish the diet day with a creamy *strawberry shake,* which you make by blending one cup fresh strawberries, one cup skim milk, one-quarter cup club soda and some crushed ice. Blend and serve at once.

As you see, this is a blender diet. Don't try to concoct these thick shakes without one—it won't work well.

Beef Stew Diet

A hearty, winter weight-loss program, the Beef Stew Diet is easy on the budget and, once you've laid in your supply of stew, requires only five minutes preparation time per meal.

All meals are exactly the same—including breakfast. Three times a day, you are allowed to have as much as you want of beef stew. It just depends on your appetite!

Follow any standard recipe for this dish. I include only carrots for the vegetable—they're all more or less alike, give or take a few herb seasonings. Prepare at least three or four pounds of stew (this amount should see you through about three diet days); so that all you have to do at mealtime is heat and eat.

These are protein-packed meals so filling that you won't feel hungry at all. And if you find the idea of beef stew for breakfast unfamiliar, try it before you reject the diet for this reason. On a cold winter morning, a bowl of hot beef stew is at least as satisfying as a cup of dry cereal!

Along with meals, you may have water, artificially sweetened soft drinks and unlimited quantities of black coffee or plain tea.

The Salad Smash

Salad buffs are a special breed. Keep your steak, your ice cream parfaits, your lasagna and your cherry cheesecake; the salad lover will turn a nose up at these gourmet treats in favor of a big bowl of cool and crispy greens topped with a favorite dressing. If you can identify with this person, you're probably not overweight. But if you do love salads and also need to shed a few pounds, consider my Salad Smash, a weight-off plan that will reduce you by about five pounds in three days.

Meals consist solely of salads, three different kinds per day.

Breakfast: Have a fresh fruit salad, one whole cupful, chilled and garnished with peppermint leaves. Prepare enough for two or three servings. Then store what you don't eat for the following day. Include orange and grapefruit sections, cantaloupe or melon chunks, green grapes, apple and pineapple (mix your own favorites). You may also have black coffee or tea.

Lunch: A tossed green salad, your choice of ingredients from among these: bibb, Boston, or iceberg lettuce, romaine or escarole, endive, onion, green pepper, celery, carrots and tomatoes. Season with two teaspoons of your favorite dressing.

Dinner: A large shrimp bowl . . . ¼ pound of shrimp, cooked and chilled, served on a bed of lettuce. You may have a moderate amount of cocktail sauce.

The Cheese and Tomato Slimmer

This is your basic crash diet—essentially, two foods: plump, ripe red tomatoes and American or cheddar cheese. If you've a lover of grilled cheese and tomato sandwiches, as I am, this is the quickie diet for you.

Breakfast on the C&T Slimmer is one slice of American cheese or an equivalent amount of cheddar, grilled on a slice of whole wheat or protein-bread toast.

Lunch is nearly the same, except that at noon you may have two slices of cheese, plus three slices of tomato, on your open-faced grilled sandwich.

Dinner does something entirely different with the same ingredients. You are permitted two tomatoes and two ounces of crumbled cheese. Prepare by scooping out the insides of the tomatoes, leaving a thick shell. Fill each tomato with half the cheese. Sprinkle with a tiny bit of bread crumb and a dab of butter and grill under the broiler until the cheese has completely melted within the tomato shells. Serve hot.

With each meal, you may have either black coffee or plain tea. If you wish you may sweeten these with an artificial sweetener.

The Peanut Butter Diet

We all know peanut butter addicts. Thick, gooey, finger-licking, lip-smacking peanut butter—the only argument you can have with a true peanut butter lover is, "creamy or chunky?" Here then, for aficionados, the diet suprème, a weight loss plan that allows (almost) nothing but the mouthwatering butter of the humble peanut.

Breakfast is one tablespoon of peanut butter on a slice of toast. You must have either whole wheat or protogen bread, both more thinning than other kinds.

Lunch is almost the same. You may, however, add two slices of fried bacon to your peanut-butter sandwich. Still only one slice of bread and one tablespoon of peanut butter.

Dinner is . . . you guessed it, peanut butter! More and more of the same: two slices of bread, again whole wheat or protogen, and two tablespoonsful of your favorite PB brand. Top with cucumber slices, lettuce or bean sprouts.

With each meal you may have coffee or tea, served hot or cold (no milk or cream), water or a calorie-free soft drink.

And, by the way, on this diet, the choice of creamy or chunky is *completely* up to you.

The Cream Soup Diet

You may have three bowls of rich cream soup every day on this diet, which will help you take off five pounds in three days if you stick to these few delectable rules.

For breakfast, lunch and dinner, you may take your choice of the following soups:

cream of asparagus
cream of celery
cream of chicken
cream of tomato
cream of potato

Soups must be made with skim milk, and you may have one cup per meal, accompanied by two slices of unsalted melba toast.

If you're particularly fond of one soup, asparagus for example, you may have that soup exclusively for every meal of your diet—all contain approximately the same calorie values, and so long as you limit yourself to one cup, you'll reduce on schedule.

Garnish soups with chopped parsley, chopped chives or herbs and spices to taste.

The Can't-Live-Without-Sweets Diet

How many dieters' firm resolve has been shattered just at the crucial moment by an uncontrollable lust for something sweet? Personally, I'd hate to count how many diets I've broken because I just couldn't get through another day without a piece of cake, some ice cream or a bit of candy. And I know I'm not alone in this folly. So many of my friends reported an irresistible desire for sweets that a few years ago I devised a diet plan which would allow an individual to lose weight (at least two pounds a week) while satisfying a passion for sweets. I call it the Can't-Live-Without-Sweets Diet; it's for those poor souls who can't bear the thought of being deprived of this particular pleasure.

You can follow this seven-day weight loss plan without including the daily allotment of sweets and lose at an even quicker rate. This is basically a balanced, low-calorie diet which limits you to 900 calories per day. At that rate, you can expect to lose three pounds per week. Opting to include your daily sweet, however, the regime still keeps intake to approximately 1100 calories. Just watch the pounds melt away as you have the last laugh over a sumptuous piece of devil's food cake!

THE CAN'T-LIVE-WITHOUT-SWEETS MENUS

This is, as I've said, a seven-day plan, with seven basic menus. Easy to follow, they require little preparation time, and are relatively lenient on the budget. Following are a week's worth of menus, Monday to Sunday.

Monday

Breakfast
1 small apple
1 slice dry white toast
½ cup creamed cottage cheese
coffee or tea

Lunch
4 oz. lean hamburger
lettuce and tomato salad
1 dill pickle
1 small banana
coffee or tea

Dinner
½ grapefruit
3½ oz. broiled chicken breast
1 cup cooked chopped spinach
1 cup cooked beets
coffee or tea

Tuesday

Breakfast
½ grapefruit
1 egg
1 slice dry toast
coffee or tea

Lunch
1 small can water-packed tuna
1 cup lettuce
½ cucumber
1 medium tomato
1 slice white bread
coffee or tea

Dinner
4 oz. broiled calves liver
1 cup broccoli spears
1 cup cooked carrots
½ cup rice
coffee or tea

Wednesday

Breakfast
1 large orange
1 egg
1 slice dry toast
coffee or tea

Lunch
3½ oz. broiled chicken
  breast
2 raw carrots
2 celery stalks
tossed green salad
coffee or tea

Dinner
1 cup steamed eggplant
1 cup stewed tomatoes
½ cup sautéed mushrooms on . . .
1 slice toast
coffee or tea

Thursday

Breakfast
1 cup unsweetened
  grapefruit juice
1 cup dry high-protein
  cereal with . . .
½ cup skim milk
  and . . .
½ banana, sliced
coffee or tea

Lunch
1 egg salad sandwich
lettuce and tomato salad
coffee or tea

Dinner
4 oz. lean hamburger
1 cup broccoli spears
½ cup green peas
1 cup lettuce and endive salad
coffee or tea

Friday

Breakfast
1 oz. cheddar cheese
1 small apple
1 cup skim milk

Lunch
4 canned sardines
½ cup creamed cottage
  cheese
lettuce and tomato salad
3 saltines
coffee or tea

Dinner

3 oz. baked flounder
½ cup rice
1 cup cooked spinach
1 cup yellow squash
coffee or tea

Saturday

Breakfast

1 cup cooked oatmeal
1 cup orange juice
coffee or tea

Lunch

1 cup Waldorf salad (apple, celery, walnut)
3 slices melba toast
coffee or tea

Dinner

4 oz. round steak, lean cut
1 small baked potato with 2 tsp. sour cream
½ cup sautéed mushrooms
½ cup brussels sprouts
tossed green salad
coffee or tea

Sunday

Breakfast

1 cup unsweetened grapefruit juice
2 strips bacon
1 egg
1 slice dry toast
coffee or tea

Lunch

4 oz. lean hamburger
1 medium tomato
tossed green salad
coffee or tea

Dinner

½ lb. chicken chow mein
½ cup rice
coffee or tea

Now for the fun! In addition to the foods listed on the menus, you may choose ONE item from the list below each day—remember, just ONE of these sweet treats per day! (Please note that five gingersnap cookies, for example, counts as ONE sweet food. You may in this case have five cookies. Because of the caloric variations from item to item, you must limit yourself to exactly the quantity specified.)

Choose ONE item daily from the list below:

- ½ slice devil's food cake with icing
- 1 slice sponge cake
- 1 slice angel's food cake
- 1 plain doughnut
- 4 butter cookies
- 2 chocolate chip cookies
- 5 gingersnap cookies
- 1 large oatmeal with raisin cookie
- 3 shortbread cookies
- 4 vanilla wafers
- 1 fruit-filled turnover
- ½ cup ice milk
- ⅓ cup ice cream
- ½ cup sherbet
- 1 cup fruit-flavored gelatin
- 2 tbsp. jam or marmalade
- 5 plain or chocolate caramels
- 2 chocolate cream-filled candies
- 5 marshmallows

And that's not all . . . you may, during the course of the day—every day—have TWO lollipops (size one inch square by ¼ inch thick) *or* TWO equivalent-sized hard sucking candies.

Not permitted: Butter, mayonnaise, catsup and other condiments; also, anything *not* included on the preceding menus and lists.

Permitted: unlimited quantities of water, calorie-free soft drinks, bouillon, black coffee or tea.

Diet tips: If you know you have an activity-filled weekend ahead, with dinners out or company coming to your own house—which means lots of desserts, lots of temptation—you may eliminate your daily sweet for one or two days during the week in order to double up over the weekend. Don't, for example, have any sweets on Tuesday and Thursday, then have two on Friday and Saturday! You may still have only the sweets listed above, but twice as much seems like a party to dieters.

I use the lollipop/candy allowance as a pacifier. Just when I feel my sweets craving making its presence felt, I pop a lollipop into my mouth. Sticky and sweet, it lasts for a very long 10 minutes, and placates me perfectly.

The Low-calorie Health Diet

Here, at last, my own super-sensible pounds-off program, a trustworthy diet I've stayed with for a week and lived on for a month. It's nutritionally balanced for good health, which means you get all the necessary proteins, carbos and fats for long-range dieting if flab is out of control. Essentially, this is a low-calorie plan which limits your intake to between 1000 and 1200 calories per day. If you stick with it, and don't cheat, weight loss is approximately three or four pounds per week. The simple menus are ones I really enjoy, but you should feel free to substitute "similar" foods for my choices (for example, fish for chicken; broccoli for spinach). Just make sure that substitute foods contain approximately the same calorie value.

Eat three times a day and at the same time each day. You may *not* snack between meals, but you may fill up on unlimited quantities of water, club soda, beef or chicken bouillon or broth and calorie-free carbonated beverages. And don't forget that daily multivitamin.

Monday

Breakfast
1 medium orange
½ cup cooked cereal
  with ½ pat butter
  and ½ cup skim
  milk
coffee or tea

Lunch
tuna fish sandwich (made
  with 1 tsp. mayonnaise
  and ½ small can tuna)
scallions
tomato wedges with 1 tsp.
  dressing
1 small pear
coffee or tea

Dinner
1 cup beef consommé with scallions
1 lamb chop
1 cup spinach
½ cup corn niblets
coffee or tea

Tuesday

Breakfast
1 cup strawberries
2 oz. cottage cheese
1 slice dry toast
coffee or tea

Lunch
4 oz. hamburger on ½ bun
spinach and mushroom sal-
    ad with 2 tsp. oil and
    vinegar dressing
¼ cantaloupe with lemon
coffee or tea

Dinner
½ grapefruit
1 medium pork chop
1 cup brussels sprouts with
    1 pat butter
tossed green salad with lemon
    dressing
1 small roll
coffee or tea

Wednesday

Breakfast
½ grapefruit
1 poached egg on . . .
1 slice toast
coffee or tea

Lunch
1 broiled chicken breast
    with rosemary
escarole salad with 2 tsp.
    French dressing
carrot sticks
celery stalks
1 medium apple
coffee or tea

Dinner
4 oz. broiled striped bass with
    lemon slices
1 cup brussels sprouts with 1 pat
    butter
½ cup rice
romaine lettuce salad with 1 tsp.
    French dressing
½ cup ice milk
coffee or tea

Thursday

Breakfast
½ cup orange juice
¾ cup dry cereal with
   ½ cup blueberries
   and ½ cup skim
   milk
coffee or tea

Lunch
1 cup beef consommé with
   chives
4 oz. London broil slices
1 cup broccoli with 1 pat
   butter
½ cup pineapple
coffee or tea

Dinner
4 oz. broiled chicken breast
½ cup rice
½ cup cøoked carrots
1 cup summer squash
no-calorie gelatin dessert
coffee or tea

Friday

Breakfast
1 medium orange
2 broiled kippers on ...
1 slice dry toast
coffee or tea

Lunch
1 broiled frank with American cheese on thin sliced
   wheat bread
½ cup sauerkraut
1 sour pickle
coffee or tea

Dinner
4 oz. broiled scallops
1 cup steamed watercress with
   1 pat butter
½ cup corn
1 broiled tomato with herbs
1 small roll
coffee or tea

Saturday

Breakfast
1 cup orange juice
1 mushroom omelette
(made with 1 egg
and 4 oz. mushroom
coffee or tea

Lunch
1 scoop tuna fish salad
(made with ½ small can
tuna, 1 stalk celery, 1
tsp. mayonnaise)
2 tbsp. cottage cheese
8 asparagus spears with tarragon vinegar
no-calorie gelatin dessert
coffee or tea

Dinner
¼ cantaloupe
4 oz. roast turkey
½ cup mashed potatoes
1 cup string beans
½ cup beets
coffee or tea

Sunday

Breakfast
½ cantaloupe
2 oz. cottage cheese
2 slices melba toast
coffee or tea

Lunch
1 turkey sandwich with 1
tsp. mayonnaise on thin
sliced white bread
pickled string bean and
onion salad
coffee or tea

Dinner
4 oz. broiled chopped steak
4 oz. mushrooms, sautéed in 1 tbsp.
butter
tomato and cucumber salad with
vinegar dressing
1 slice whole wheat bread
1 medium apple
coffee or tea

CORINNE'S LOW-CARBOHYDRATE DIET RECIPES

The major problem with any low-carbohydrate diet, at least in my experience, is boredom. After about a week or two of low-carb eating, I find myself craving a slice of bread, a sweet to nibble on, a bit of pie crust on which to pile my permitted creamy desserts.

My version of a low-carbohydrate diet is therefore very simple: it consists of all the usual fare, but also includes bread, cookies, candy and other "forebidden" foods. Not ordinary goodies, but made from recipes carefully devised with a low-carbohydrate-dieting friend.

Here they are, for your eating pleasure, complete with carbohydrate gram counts . . .

Real Yeast Bread

1 tbsp. active dry yeast	1 tsp. sugar substitute (optional)
2 tbsp. warm water	1½ cups sifted gluten flour
2 tbsp. melted butter or margarine	½ cup sifted soy flour
½ tsp. salt	½ cup toasted wheat germ cereal

Soften yeast for about 10 minutes in two tablespoons of warm water. Add one cup of warm water, butter or margarine, salt and sugar substitute to yeast; stir. Combine flours with wheat germ and add to yeast mixture. Mix well, then knead dough for about 15 minutes. Shape into loaf and put in nine-inch loaf pan. Cover and let rise in a warm place until dough doubles in bulk. Bake at 350°F until golden brown (about 50–60 minutes). Let cool on rack before slicing. Makes one large loaf.

Entire recipe . . . . .122.2 carbohydrate grams
One slice (¼ inch thick) . . . .3.4 carbohydrate grams

Soy Loaf

4 large eggs	¾ cup water
1 cup sifted soy flour	1 tsp. salt
2 tsp. baking powder	2 tbsp. melted butter, margarine or oil

Separate eggs. Beat yolks until lemon colored. Combine flours with baking powder and salt. Add water, egg yolks and butter, margarine or oil. Mix well to make a smooth batter. Beat egg whites until very stiff, then fold into batter. Pour or spoon mixture into a greased nine-inch loaf pan. Bake at 375°F until golden brown (about 45–50 minutes). Let cool before serving. Makes one large loaf.

Entire recipe . . . . 40.7 carbohydrate grams
One slice (½ inch thick) . . . .2.3 carbohydrate grams

Soy Nut Loaf

7 large eggs	⅛ cup nonfat dry milk
1 cup sifted soy flour	¼ cup chopped walnuts
½ cup heavy cream	1 tbsp. oil
½ tsp. salt	1 tbsp. soy flour
1 tsp. sugar substitute (optional)	

Separate eggs. Beat yolks until lemon colored. Blend in flour slowly—⅓ cup at a time—using a wire whisk. Beat in heavy cream, salt, sugar substitute and dry milk. Stir in walnuts. Beat egg whites until very stiff, then fold into mixture carefully. Pour or spoon batter into a nine-inch loaf pan which has been greased with one tablespoon of oil and coated with one tablespoon of flour.

Bake at 350°F until golden brown (about 50–60 minutes). Let cool before serving. Makes one large loaf.

Entire recipe . . . . .66.6 carbohydrate grams
One slice (½ inch thick) . . . .3.7 carbohydrate grams

Cheese Biscuits

¾ cup sifted gluten flour	2 tbsp. butter or margarine
6 tbsp. soy flour	½ cup sour cream
1 tsp. baking powder	3 tbsp. grated sharp cheese
½ tsp. baking soda	½ tsp. sugar substitute (optional)
½ tsp. salt	

Sift flours with baking powder, soda and salt. Cut in butter or margarine. Add sour cream, cheese and sugar substitute; blend thoroughly. Shape into 18 balls. Put on a baking sheet and flatten balls with fork. Bake at 375°F until golden brown (about 30 minutes). Makes 18 biscuits.

Entire recipe . . . . .59.8 carbohydrate grams
One biscuit . . . . .3.3 carbohydrate grams

Oatmeal Muffins

3 tbsp. oatmeal cereal	1 tsp. baking powder
½ cup heavy cream	½ tsp. salt
1 large egg	1 tsp. melted butter, margarine or oil
½ cup sifted gluten flour	

Soak oatmeal in heavy cream for 15 minutes. Beat egg and add to oatmeal. Add flour resifted with baking powder and salt. Blend well. Grease muffin tins with butter, margarine or oil. Half fill 12 tins with batter. Bake at 325°F until golden brown (about 40 minutes). Makes 12 muffins.

Entire recipe . . . . .44.7 carbohydrate grams
One muffin . . . . .3.7 carbohydrate grams

Pie Crust

½ cup sifted gluten flour
¼ cup sifted soy flour
¼ tsp. salt

4 tbsp. butter or margarine
1 tbsp. ice water

Resift flours with salt. Cut in butter or margarine and mix well. Add ice water and blend thoroughly to make a smooth ball. Roll out thin and line a nine-inch pie plate or tin. Prick crust evenly with fork and bake in 375°F oven until browned. Makes one large pie crust.

Entire recipe ....40.2 carbohydrate grams
One section (12 per pie crust) ...... 3.3 carbohydrate grams

Nutty Pie Crust

½ lb. shelled Brazil nuts
2 tbsp. butter
2 tbsp. gluten flour

1 tsp. liquid sugar substitute
1 tsp. cinnamon

Grind nuts in blender. Combine nuts with remaining ingredients and mix well. Pat mixture into a nine-inch pie plate or tin and bake 10–15 minutes at 350°F. Chill before filling. Makes one pie crust.

Entire recipe ....32.9 carbohydrate grams
One section (12 per pie crust) ......2.7 carbohydrate grams

Peanut Butter Cookies

½ cup melted butter or vegetable oil
2 tsp. granulated sugar substitute
2 eggs
6 tbsp. peanut butter

2 tbsp. water
¾ cup sifted gluten flour
½ tsp. salt

Beat butter or oil with sugar substitute and eggs. Add peanut butter, water, flour and salt. Mix well. Drop by teaspoonfuls onto a greased cookie sheet; flatten with fork if necessary. Bake in 350°F oven until browned. Makes about 24 cookies.

Entire recipe . . . . .62.6 carbohydrate grams
One cookie . . . . .2.6 carbohydrate grams

Almond Cookies

½ cup sifted gluten flour
1 tsp. granulated sugar substitute
½ cup chopped almonds
½ tsp. vanilla flavoring
½ tsp. almond flavoring
light cream

Combine all ingredients, adding enough light cream to lightly moisten mixture. Shape into 18 balls. Place on a greased cookie sheet and bake at 400°F for about 15–20 minutes. Let cool. Makes 18 cookies.

Entire recipe . . . . .43.7 carbohydrate grams
One cookie . . . . .2.4 carbohydrate grams

Chocolate Whip

1 oz. unsweetened grated chocolate
⅓ cup water
⅔ cup heavy cream
dash salt
1 tbsp. unflavored gelatin
¼ cup water
2 large eggs
2 tsp. vanilla flavoring
dash sugar substitute

Combine chocolate, one-third cup of water, cream and salt in top of a double boiler; heat, stirring, until chocolate melts. Soften gelatin in cold water. Add to heated chocolate mixture and stir over low heat until gelatin dissolves. Remove from heat. Separate eggs. Beat yolks until lemon colored and add to chocolate mixture. Return to heat and stir gently in top of double boiler until mixture thickens. Remove from heat and stir in vanilla and sugar substitute. Beat egg white until very stiff and fold into mixture. Spoon into individual serving dishes and chill until set. Makes 4–6 servings.

Entire recipe . . . . 13.9 carbohydrate grams
One serving (4 servings per recipe) . . 3.5 carbohydrate grams
One serving (6 servings per recipe) . . 2.3 carbohydrate grams

Rum Custard

1 egg, beaten	½ tsp. sugar substitute (op-
½ cup heavy cream	tional)
½ tsp. rum liquor or	dash salt
rum flavoring	

Combine all ingredients and mix well to blend. Pour into four individual serving cups. Set cups in a pan of hot water and bake at 350°F until done (when done, a knife inserted into center of custard will come out clean). Makes four servings.

Entire recipe . . . . 4.2 carbohydrate grams
One serving . . . . 1.1 carbohydrate grams

Nut Fudge

6 tbsp. peanut butter	½ tsp. vanilla flavoring
½ cup regular nonfat	¾ tsp. liquid sugar substi-
dry milk	tute
1½ tbsp. unsweetened	1 tbsp. heavy cream
dry cocoa	¼ cup broken walnuts
⅛ tsp. salt	

Combine all ingredients, except heavy cream and walnuts. Mash well. Add cream slowly, mixing thoroughly. Put mixture on a piece of waxed paper and sprinkle on nuts. Knead until nuts are blended in. Cover with waxed paper and roll out to half-inch thickness. Cut into 16 one-inch squares. Makes 16 pieces.

Entire recipe . . . . 41.9 carbohydrate grams
One piece . . . . 2.6 carbohydrate grams

Marzipan

4 oz. blanched al-
    monds
½ cup unsweetened
    grated coconut
⅓ cup regular nonfat
    dry milk
¼ cup heavy cream
dash salt

1 tsp. vanilla flavoring
½ tsp. almond flavoring
2 tbsp. liquid sugar substi-
    tute
food coloring (optional)

Put almonds and coconut in blender; blend at high
speed to flour consistency. Add dry milk and cream,
and mix well. Add salt, flavorings and sugar substitute
gradually to taste. If desired, add a few drops food coloring and mix color in evenly. Let stand for one hour.
Shape as desired; let dry overnight. Wrap and store in
refrigerator. Makes about 30 pieces.

Entire recipe . . . . 46.7 carbohydrate grams
One piece . . . . 1.5 carbohydrate grams

Brazil Balls

2 tbsp. peanut butter
2 tbsp. cream cheese
¼ cup regular nonfat
    dry milk
1 tsp. heavy cream

6 tbsp. chopped Brazil nuts
dash sugar substitute (op-
    tional)
2 tbsp. ground Brazil nuts

Combine all ingredients, except two tablespoons of
ground Brazil nuts, and mix thoroughly with fork.
Shape into 24 balls. Roll each ball in ground nuts. Chill
or freeze. Makes 24 balls.

Entire recipe . . . . 22.7 carbohydrate grams
One piece . . . . 0.9 carbohydrate grams

NUTRITION AND DIETING

If dieting is a short-term project, proper nutrition should be, for those who value their health as well as their newfound slimness, a lifelong goal. I promise you, you won't be able to keep that extra weight off until you resolve to start eating right. And what does that mean? Proper nutrition simply means examining your regular diet and, where necessary, juggling and exchanging certain foods so that what you end up with is the *proper* balance of carbohydrates, fats, proteins, vitamins, minerals and water. For most people, alterations are minor, although for some people, the switch to a healthful pattern of eating will mean changing habits of a lifetime. Good health is worth the effort.

Let me tell you what a difference proper nutrition can make. About three years ago, Sally, who is a New York friend of mine, went on Dr. Atkins' Diet to rid herself of 20 extra pounds, which had taken form on her as a spare tire, saddlebags and championship arms. After two months of faithful dieting, she succeeded in losing all her flab. Sally was delirious to be back to her normal weight (even below it!), and friends told her that her figure never looked so good. A month after that, Sally's figure still looked great, but she looked terrible. Tired, dragged out, slow-moving . . . we really started to worry, but Sally insisted she wasn't ill.

Late one night I received a phone call from Sally. She was on her way to the airport, headed for sunny Florida. Doctor's orders. Admitting to herself that she felt horrid, she'd taken herself over to the doctor's office that afternoon for a physical. She got that, too, but she received an angry lecture from her doctor, a man not noted for his sweet temperament. He was appalled at Sally's diet, which in those days consisted of coffee and doughnut for breakfast, cottage cheese and coffee for lunch, and an Italian hero from the corner delicatessan for dinner. What, asked the irritated doctor, was she trying to do—kill herself? He gave her a mimeographed diet, which he commanded her to follow, and told her to go away and rest. Meekly, Sally obeyed. Two weeks later, she returned to New York, a disciple of proper nutrition—and orange juice. She now eats sanely and regularly, and I'll say that Sally has never looked prettier, nor seemed happier in her life.

Of course, you needn't resort to a physical collapse to learn about nutrition. By far the best teacher is a preventive education. The facts are simple; the basics are easy to remember; and, in fact, good nutrition is one of the easiest things in the world for people to attain.

There are five basic rules of nutrition. Anything more is just refinement or commentary on these guidelines. Follow these few rules and I can practically guarantee that you'll be eating well and maintaining your weight and good health without additional effort.

The five rules are: (1) Limit the number of calories you intake. (2) Eat lots of protein. (3) Limit the amount of fat you consume and keep sugar consumption to a minimum. (4) Select foods from the Four Basic Food Groups each day. (5) Get enough vitamins and minerals in your diet.

I'll explain each of these points further . . .

1. *Limit your calories:* You can maintain your desirable weight by intaking *only* the number of calories your body needs to function. If you consume more calories than you require, you'll gain weight, and conversely, when you don't get enough, the scales will drop. The number of calories you require is listed in the Caloric Maintenance Chart on page 159. Remember, however, that individuals differ, so that this estimate—though based on tabulated norms and averages—may be inaccurate for you. You can pretty well figure your calorie needs by doing a little at-home experimenting: Begin with the figure given on the Chart. If, at the end of a week, you find that you've *gained* weight, then *decrease* the calorie total by 100 calories per day. Try *that*

CALORIC MAINTENANCE CHART

	DESIRABLE WEIGHT	18-35 YEARS	35-55 YEARS	55-75 YEARS
WOMEN	99	1,700	1,500	1,300
	110	1,850	1,650	1,400
	121	2,000	1,750	1,550
	128	2,100	1,900	1,600
	132	2,150	1,950	1,650
	143	2,300	2,050	1,800
	154	2,400	2,150	1,850
	165	2,550	2,300	1,950
MEN	110	2,200	1,950	1,650
	121	2,400	2,150	1,850
	132	2,550	2,300	1,950
	143	2,700	2,400	2,050
	154	2,900	2,600	2,200
	165	3,100	2,800	2,400
	176	3,250	2,950	2,500
	187	3,300	3,100	2,600

*Based on moderate activity. If your life is very active, add 50 calories; if your life is sedentary, subtract 75 calories.

quota for a week. If your weight remains stable, you may rely on this as your caloric requirement. Be patient; adjust the figure up or down until you arrive at a number that designates exactly how many calories you can consume to remain at your present weight.

I suggest monitoring your calories for about a month. At the end of that time, you'll have an accurate feeling for the amount of food you should be eating each day. Though it seems like tedious business, that month may be the most valuable one you'll ever spend on your figure. Knowing how much you can safely eat, being able to "feel" when you've overstepped your limits, being able to judge types of foods and portions in terms of your weight may be the knowledge that will keep you from ever having to diet again!

2. *Eat lots of protein:* Protein, as you know by now, is one of the most important nutrients, essential for cell repair and tissue growth and rebuilding. Make sure you get lots of it, in the form of meat, fish and poultry, and also from other more uncommon protein sources such as cottage cheese, nuts and fortified skim milk. Protein is essential in the maintenance of good health.

3. *Limit fat and sugar consumption:* The Intersociety Commission on Heart Disease recommends that your total fat intake be limited to less than 35% of your total calorie intake daily. Monitor yourself. Go easy on butter, margarine, heavy cream, fatty meats and fish; if you include one high-fat dish on your menu, don't have two. Balance foods so that they aren't too weighted in favor of any nutrient. By the same token, foods with a high sugar content—sugars, syrups and sweet baked goods— should be limited, too. Use your common sense. You don't have to remove these foods from your diet altogether; just don't go overboard with items that have a high-calorie price tag.

4. *Select foods from the Four Basic Food Groups:* I rely on those old nutrition charts (remember them from grade school?) to tell me how to plan menus. They describe four basic food groups, and if you make sure to select foods from *each* of these groups every day, you'll be doing just fine—your menus will be nutritionally

balanced, as well as providing interest and variety for your palate. The four basic food groups are:

Milk and milk products: This group includes whole and skim milk; cheese and cheese products; yogurt; butter; cream.

Vegetables and fruits: All green and yellow vegetables and all fruits are included in this group.

Meat, fish, poultry, eggs: Included in this group are all types of meat, fish, poultry, eggs, dried beans and peas (legumes).

Grain products and bread: All grain products such as bread, cereal, cakes, cookies, and pasta are included in this group.

If you include foods from each of these groups every day, your nutritional needs will take care of themselves. A balanced diet means exactly *that*—a balanced selection from all four groups.

5. *Get enough vitamins and minerals:* These nutrients, though calorie-free and organically different from proteins, carbohydrates and fats, are essential to your good health and well being—just as important as other types of nutrients. Following is a brief primer on vitamins and minerals. Read carefully. Get to know which vitamins are contained in which common foods, so that getting a balance becomes like second nature.

VITAMINS, MINERALS, WATER AND THE "MAGICAL" DIET

VITAMINS

Vitamins are organic food substances that play an important role in human nutrition. Vitamins don't contain calories themselves, but their presence in the body is vital to regular metabolic processes; in other words, they help the body to break down and use foods and assist in the formation of bone and tissue. The body does not manufacture vitamins; we get them from the foods we eat, and if you're wondering about vitamin pills and whether you really need them or not, the answer is simple. If you're getting all your required vitamins from the foods you eat, no supplement should be necessary, except in unusual cases. When your diet is not nutritionally balanced (as in the case of some weight-loss diets), a multiple vitamin supplement may be prescribed by your doctor.

The following basic vitamins are contained in the foods we eat. Each vitamin is helpful to the body in a particular way, so it's important to include a source of each in your regular meal planning.

Vitamin A: This vitamin is believed necessary to the normal functioning of the skin cells, and, your ability to see in the dark depends on taking in enough vitamin A—a deficiency causes a condition called "night blindness." Vitamin A is contained in egg yolks, butter, cheese, carrots, leafy greens, dark green and deep yellow vegetables such as broccoli and turnip, fish and fish oils, pumpkin, sweet potatoes, winter squash, apricots, cantaloupe.

Vitamin B_1 (thiamine): In children, this is one of

the important growth vitamins and may even play a part in determining children's ability to learn. In adults, vitamin B_1 is one of the essential "nerve vitamins" which promote the smooth functioning of the nervous system and health of the muscular systems. Lack of vitamin B_1 is believed to be a cause of mental depression, and so it's called the "morale vitamin." This vitamin is plentiful in natural foods, whole grain cereals and breads, "enriched" breads, wheat germ, brewers' yeast, bakers' yeast, dried beans, peas, lean pork, heart, kidney, liver and all kinds of lean meat.

Vitamin B_2 (riboflavin): Riboflavin deficiency causes visual disturbances, such as increased sensitivity to light, gradual loss of vision and cataracts. This vitamin is so plentiful in the foods we commonly eat, that deficiencies are indeed rare. Some good sources of vitamin B_2 are leafy vegetables, eggs and egg whites, liver, kidney and other organ meats, lean meats, vegetables, milk, cottage cheese and bread.

Niacin (nicotinic acid): Like most of the B-complex vitamins, niacin is vital to the normal functioning of the nervous system. It also plays a part in the maintenance of the health of the skin—a niacin deficiency causes conditions such as pellagra and dermatitis. Rich sources of niacin are lean meats, poultry, fish, yeast, legumes, peanuts and peanut butter, enriched bread and fortified milk.

Vitamin C (ascorbic acid): Vitamin C, about which so much has been written in recent years, is one of the most important vitamins for good health. This vitamin helps to maintain the health of the connective tissues and also aids in forming red blood cells and preventing hemorrhage. It is believed to be an infection-fighting vitamin, and is therefore used by some in treating and preventing the common cold. Vitamin C deficiency results in a disease called scurvy, which is characterized by bleeding gums, weakened teeth, and general fragility of the blood vessels. Since smoking destroys large amounts of vitamin C in the body, smokers are advised to supplement their diet with vitamin C or to eat bigger than usual portions of the following high-C foods: fresh fruits and vegetables, including all citrus fruits, cantaloupe, strawberries, broccoli, brussels sprouts, raw cabbage, collards, green and sweet red peppers, mustard and turnip greens, tomatoes.

Vitamin D: Vitamin D is the "healthy bones" vitamin, and if you live in a sunny clime you may not even need any additional sources of D, since the sun acts to convert certain skin oils directly to vitamin D. Most of us need to get vitamin D in food, and fish is one very good source. Salmon, sardines, herring, cod, halibut and tuna are rich in vitamin D; milk is often fortified with vitamin D.

Vitamin E: Data about vitamin E is inconclusive, but it is believed that the vitamin may promote fertility in humans, as it does in certain laboratory animals. Vitamin E is plentiful in wheat germ, vegetable oils and polyunsaturated fats.

Vitamin K: Vitamin K is necessary in the process of blood clotting, and is plentiful in kelp, lettuce, spinach, alfalfa and leafy green vegetables.

These are the primary vitamins; there are other vitamins, but the importance of these substances has not thus far been conclusively established. Let me say once more that if you are eating a wholesome, balanced diet, all your vitamin needs will be met without the need for supplementary pills or capsules. Before you embark on any weight-loss program, ask your doctor about taking a multiple-vitamin supplement; he may want to recommend one that is high in a particular vitamin.

MINERALS

Minerals must also be included in your diet for vitality. They're essential for metabolism and keep bones, blood and teeth strong and healthy. The primary minerals are:

Calcium: Pay special attention to calcium in meal planning, since this mineral is present in very *few* foods. Calcium, which keeps the skeleton and bones strong, is contained in milk and dairy products and bone meal. Lack of calcium in one's diet may lead to degeneration of the spine, softening and cracking of the bones and arthritis.

Iodine: Iodine is important in maintaining and regulating the body's metabolism since it is an important element in thyroxin, the hormone produced by the thyroid or "metabolism" gland. Iodine is present in seafood, iodized salt and mushrooms.

Iron: Iron is necessary to the formation of hemoglobin, which transports oxygen to the organs and tissues of the body—that's why people say that iron enriches the blood. The best source of iron is liver. Lean beef and other organ meats as well as oysters, shellfish and some leafy green vegetables supply iron to the body.

Other minerals, including sodium, potassium, magnesium, phosphorus and zinc, are also necessary, although for many of these the exact amount required by the body has not been established. Again, if you are eating a well-balanced diet, including foods from all the basic food groups, these minerals will automatically be included in your daily menus.

WATER

Water is a nutrient, more abundant in the body than any other. Water, which makes up about two-thirds of the body's weight, may be said to be the most important nutritive element, since without it digestion, absorption, circulation and excretion could not take place. Every function of the body depends on water.

Under normal circumstances, most adults lose three quarts daily through perspiration and excretion; in hotter climates, or with more strenuous exercise, more water is lost. Most of the water we give off is replaced by that contained in the foods we eat—nearly every food contains this valuable nutrient. But it is recommended by most doctors and nutritionists that we drink extra liquids, either water, beverages, soups or juices.

It is important to note that the considerations of nutrition discussed here apply in situations where health is normal, and where no unusual medical problems exist. Special conditions such as an abnormally high cholesterol level, hypoglycemia, diabetes, heart or kidney disease or disorders of the liver demand exclusive attention, and the analysis that only a qualified physician or medical specialist is able to give. If you suffer from one of these problems, or from another chronic ailment, let your doctor be the best judge of your diet. He alone will be able to prescribe for you the foods demanded by your condition, those items that will help, rather than aggravate, your system.

If, however, you are in good health, do follow my five nutrition rules. They're common sense at its very wisest, and could make all the difference to your health.

One note here about cholesterol, which has been the subject of widespread discussion and sometimes-angry debate over recent years. One of the most furious attacks against low-carbohydrate and high-protein diets has been that they raise cholesterol levels in the body, and hence heighten the risk of heart disease. "Heart attack diets," these programs are called by critics. Is it true? Should cholesterol intake be limited? Eliminated altogether?

Cholesterol *per se* is no villain. It is, rather, a natural substance produced by the body and is abundant in bile produced by the liver. Cholesterol performs a very specific job: that is, to assist in the formation of adrenal hormones. The substance also appears in nerve tissue and in the brain.

As well as being produced by the body itself, cholesterol enters our bodies by way of certain foods we eat, those animal products that are extremely high in cholesterol content. Cholesterol levels may be measured by examining a blood sample, in which cholesterol milligrams are counted.

Current research indicates that there may be a link between high cholesterol levels and heart disease; excessive amounts of cholesterol in the blood seem to increase the risks of heart attack, stroke and other coronary disorders.

The best safeguard I know is a doctor's examination. As part of your pre-diet check-up, your doctor should take your cholesterol count. If your level is high (over 200 milligrams is considered too high), he may choose to put you on his own special diet to lower your cholesterol count. Cholesterol levels may be decreased with a dietary change, so follow his orders. Foods you will have to avoid are saturated fats; cholesterol-high liver, kidney, brains and sweetbreads; shellfish, including oysters, mussels, and clams; butter; cream; regular whole milk cheese, and egg yolks. The Intersociety Commission for Heart Disease recommends a daily cholesterol intake of not more than 300 milligrams.

THE LECITHIN-KELP-VINEGAR-B$_6$ DIET

Why not talk about this diet-of-the-moment right here? After all, we are on the subject of vitamins and minerals, and that's what this fad weight-loss plan is all about. Popularized in one of the women's consumer magazines, this diet depends on the "magical" properties of four natural substances, all working together to whisk pounds away, whittle inches from the body's problem areas. Does it work? Advocates swear it does. But you be the judge of that.

This diet depends on *lecithin,* a natural fat-emulsifier; *cider vinegar,* made from pure apples; *kelp,* better known as sea-spinach; and *vitamin B$_6$,* one of the powerful B-complex vitamins. Take all four of these elements and, according to this diet's fans, you'll be able to lose inches where flab has previously clung with tenacity—on hips, at the tops of thighs, on your derrière, wherever you couldn't lose before. The combination of these four ingredients just seems to loosen fat from its moorings so that it just seems to float off . . .

Follow a regular low-calorie diet—from 1000 to 1200 calories daily—and, in addition, take:

Lecithin: Lecithin, which is a fatty substance, acts itself to break up fat. Proponents of this diet believe that we do not get enough lecithin in our food to perform this function effectively, so we've got to add to our lecithin arsenal. It may be taken in granular form, sprinkled over foods or mixed with milk beverages.

Cider vinegar: The cider made from fermented apples provides your body with a bonanza of minerals, especially potassium and phosphorus, which maintain your system's good health generally as well as keeping dieting anxieties to a minimum and your good spirits up, up, up. Take one teaspoon of cider vinegar in a glass of water three times a day.

Kelp: Sea-spinach is simply a nicer name for seaweed, but what's it doing on anybody's diet? Kelp is extremely rich in iodine, which normalizes metabolism and helps you to burn foods efficiently. Kelp keeps that weight coming off—from ultra-troublesome places. Take three kelp tablets with each meal.

Vitamin B_6: Vitamin B_6 is one of the B-complex vitamins and seems to prevent excess water retention in the body, acting on water-holding sodium and water-drawing potassium to balance retention levels. Take one 50 milligram vitamin B_6 tablet daily for the duration of your diet.

For the convenience of the thousands and thousands of dieters who've flooded the nation's health food stores in search of lecithin and kelp and vitamin B_6, several pharmaceutical companies have packaged these ingredients together as one easy-to-take capsule; taking these, the dieter swallows an individual all-in-one capsule with each meal. As with any diet, check with your doctor before embarking on this popular plan—basically a low-calorie weight-loss regime, but with some fashionable magic, for those who believe.

SLIMMING WITH EXERCISE

Add exercise to your diet program, and the results will last you a lifetime. Not only will your diet work quicker, your body develop prettier lines and your health take an astounding forward leap, but exercise will help you once and for all to break the vicious cycle of fat that spells disaster for most ex-overweights. It's really the toughest problem we face: that pounds-off-pounds-on syndrome that makes thinness seem like fleeting fantasy, even when we've actually succeeded in reducing our figures!

The primary benefit of exercise—any kind of exercise—is that it puts you in touch with your body. If we're honest, we will all admit that when we're fat, we tend to cut ourselves off from our bodies. We're ashamed, angry, embarrassed and frankly disgusted by what we see in the mirror, so we protect our psyches by pretending our bodies don't belong to us. From the neck down, it's somebody else, right? That's how the vicious fat cycle begins, and appearance isn't the only thing that suffers. Health is neglected; all physical sensations, even those of sight, hearing and smell, become dulled; and sex is either ignored or forgotten. It's apparent why a serious overweight problem brings real unhappiness.

While losing weight does wonders for the morale, it may not be incentive enough to break this pattern, this negative self-image. Although you may be ardently interested in *the idea of* having a beautiful figure, actually *having and enjoying* that beautiful figure is more difficult. Even when you've lost that excess baggage, every last pound, if you don't actively enjoy your slim new body, the weight is going to go right back on. I assure you, it will.

Exercise allows you to enjoy your body. As you're bending and stretching, pushing and pulling, lifting and lowering logy old muscles you may not have budged in years, you'll suddenly experience the innate joy of really being at one with your body. It is a pleasure that rightly belongs to each of us. Perhaps for the first time in your life, you'll feel the sensuousness of stretching your spine like a graceful cat; feel the control of directing your muscles to do exactly what you want them to do; know the delight of tingling sensations in such "remote" places as your fingertips, toes, even your scalp! You'll appreciate your slim figure because it's visually attractive, but more important, because it feels so good to move your body.

Exercise is recommended for dieters because it speeds up weight loss. Any form of activity calls on the body's energy resources and burns calories, and that causes pounds to come off quicker than if you did no exercise at all. When you cut the number of calories in your diet and also utilize additional calories in mild exercise, the body is forced to mobilize an even greater amount of energy. So pounds melt away. Some nutritionists and doctors even feel that exercise improves the body's metabolic functions, making all this happen with greater efficiency.

Not only will you see quicker results, you'll witness a qualitative change in your body, too. Dieting does shrink your outline and correct outsized proportions, but cutting calories will not firm up muscles nor solidify sagging skin. You've got to exercise for a glamour-girl figure. All it takes is just a few minutes each day, a bit of diligence and discipline, but the results are definitely worth it.

Everybody knows that exercise is vital for good health. Not only will activity keep your weight down, it will also lower blood pressure significantly and keep your heart, arteries and blood vessels in tip-top shape. Remember, your heart is like any other muscle in the body; the more exercise you give it, the stronger and tougher it gets and the better it works. As you begin to exercise, the heart pumps faster (just check your pulse) and blood starts circulating rapidly throughout the whole body. That quicker pulse rate means that an even greater supply of oxygen is reaching all your vital organs and tissues, oxygen being transported by blood. With enriched supplies of life-supporting oxygen, you'll feel more vital, mentally alert and alive. I know so many dieters who've said that the tired, draggy feeling they were resigned to living with simply disappeared when they started to exercise. They felt energetic instead.

OK. The point is made. Exercise is wonderful for the body and is a special boon to dieters: it boosts morale, firms up the figure and promotes a sense of glowing vitality.

Let's be fair about it. There are certain changes exercise won't accomplish, no matter how much bending, sprinting or jumping around you do. Exercise will not alter your body structure. You've got a large frame, exercise won't transform you into a petite darling. It will, however, distribute your weight so that your body is lean and attractively well-proportioned.

Exercise will not make you taller. If you're five feet three inches with your shoes on, don't expect miracles. Exercise may, on the other hand, add an inch or two by correcting bad posture and a stoop-shouldered stance. Even if you're not tall, you'll look taller when you start carrying yourself with grace and confidence.

Exercise will not give you model-slim hips if you have a wide pelvis; if your breasts are very large or very small, exercise will not change their basic shape. What exercise will do is to tone up hips, breasts, midriff and other body areas to make muscles tight and skin smooth and taut.

All I can do at this point is to urge you to take a little time each day to start moving. Certainly, we live sedentary lives, not nearly as active as our pioneer forefathers and mothers, not even as active as our own parents. We are just plain out of the habit of making the effort. Our bodies were meant to move; we ought to give ourselves the opportunity.

What type of exercise you choose is up to you. The decision will depend on your interests, your life-style, budget and the amount of time you want to devote.

Sports such as swimming and tennis give the whole body a fine workout, and their popularity today will always provide you with an exercise partner, if you don't like to go it alone. Jogging is strenuous; I don't recommend it for anyone who isn't in perfect condition. Bicycling is another overall exercise which is fun as well as being therapeutic, and is something you can do with the whole family.

Ballet, yoga and modern dance classes attract many women, since moving to music is soothing and sexy. Classes are usually inexpensive and they're given at most Y's and local dancing schools.

I consider walking one of the best exercises in the world. Give me a pair of comfortable shoes, point me in a new direction and I'm off! Walking lets you observe the world around you as you limber up those rusty old bones, and once you hit your stride (that's when you're walking in a good, strong rhythm), you can go for hours and hours without tiring. I like a long walk after dinner on warm spring evenings and in the fall when the air is crisp and clear. Whether you're a city dweller or have the freedom of solitary country roads, walking is one of the most gratifying activities I know.

Following is a chart of various exercises, including the activity and the number of calories you'll expend per hour doing it. Remember that means calories you're burning off—the same as if you've cut them from your diet. Feel free to alternate activities. Swim one afternoon, walk the next, have a tennis game the following day . . . it doesn't matter, so long as you get in some form of exercise each day. Be faithful to it; I guarantee you'll see beautiful results within weeks.

Calorie/Exercise Chart

Activity	Calories per hour
Sitting	50
Driving a car	130
Ironing	200
Walking	200
Scrubbing floor	300
Golf	300

Gardening	340
Vigorous walking	350
Bowling	400
Tennis (doubles game)	400
Bicycling	450
Tennis (singles game)	500
Dancing	500
Skiing	600
Horseback riding	600
Jogging	600
Swimming	600
Cross-country running	640
Mountain climbing	740
Cross-country skiing	1300

For some folks, plain old bend-and-stretch routines are the easiest, most convenient way to work out. Free to choose your hour, choose your spot, wear a regulation leotard or your old nightgown, exercise to music or to the daytime soaps . . . the classic exercises are the most flexible route for many of us.

If, like me, you're too busy for outside sports and activities every day, try these routines. They're simple, and after a week or two you'll be able to breeze through them without even thinking about it. Don't be fooled. Just because these exercises aren't excruciatingly tough doesn't mean they won't do a super job of firming and tightening. Stick with this plan for two weeks, and you'll start to notice real changes in your figure. Your tummy will flatten, thighs will firm, derrière will show a perceptible lift, and you'll experience such a change in the way you feel that it will be a delightful surprise.

As with any exercise program, check with your doctor first. Explain the type of exercise program you're planning, and get the official go-ahead before you start. Don't overdo it. Especially if you haven't exercised in a long time, start out gently. Do each exercise just a few times, without straining muscles or pushing your limits. Within a short time, your stamina and capacities will increase and your whole body will become more lithe, limber—and lovely.

Deep Breathing

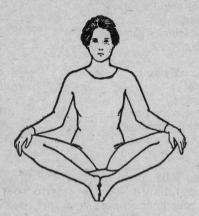

Expand your lung capacity, get your circulation moving and calm yourself down with one of the world's best exercises. Sit on the floor in a comfortable position with the soles of your feet touching, knees as close to the floor as possible. Rest your palms lightly on your knees. Keep back straight and head erect. Breathe in through your mouth, taking in as much air as you can hold into your lungs—chest and abdomen should extend and swell. Hold this breath for a count of five. Exhale through your nose, forcing the air out with a forceful whoosh.

Head Circles

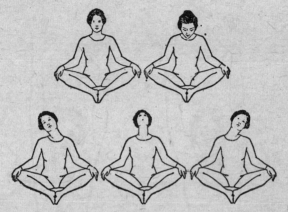

Turn your head around with this super waker-upper! Sit comfortably on the floor, with feet together, arms resting on your knees. Your spine should be straight, your shoulders relaxed and your head erect. What you're going to do is make a circle with your head: begin by dropping your head down so that your chin rests on your chest. Roll your head to the right—you should feel a stretch in your neck muscles. Continue rolling your head back, letting it drop back as far as possible. Now roll it to the left and complete the circle by rolling your head forward so that your chin again rests on your chest. Raise your head and look directly ahead.

Shoulder Raises

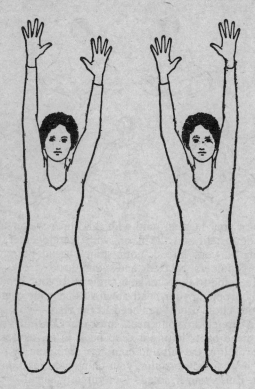

This exercise stretches the whole side of your body, your shoulders, arms and fingers—and utterly relaxes you at the same time. Begin from a kneeling position, arms down. Raise your arms above your head, palms facing front. Lifting from the shoulder, reach up to the ceiling with your right arm. Reach as high as you can. Now drop your right shoulder and lift your left shoulder, again stretching as much as possible. You should feel the muscles from your waist all the way up to your fingertips.

Easy Sit-ups

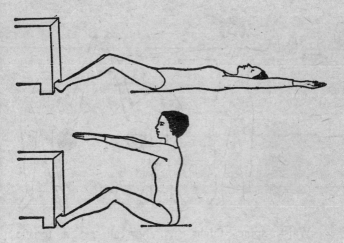

This is a modified sit-up that flattens the tummy better than any exercise I know. You'll need a heavy piece of furniture as an assist—a sofa or armchair is fine. Lie on the floor with your knees bent and feet hooked under the chair. Stretch your arms out above your head. Now sit up, pulling yourself up with your stomach muscles. Reach all the way forward with your arms. Return to your starting position.

Toe Touches

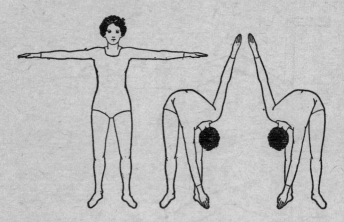

Waist, spine, thighs . . . they all get a terrific
stretching with one of my all-time favorite exercises, the
classic toe touch. Start in a standing position, feet about
18 inches apart. Extend arms to the side. Bending over
from the waist, touch your left toe with your right hand.
Return to upright position. Now touch your right toe
with your left hand. Try to keep knees perfectly
straight.

Arm Circles

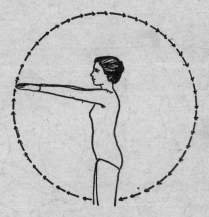

As well as exercising upper and lower arms, this easy routine is very relaxing for the whole system. Stand erect, feet slightly apart, arms resting at sides. Now raise your arms directly in front of you, palms downward. Continue lifting your arms until they're directly over your head. Lower them behind you, as far to the back as possible. Bring them to your sides, as in starting position. This movement should be a smooth circle—one continuous, sweeping gesture.

Knee Bends

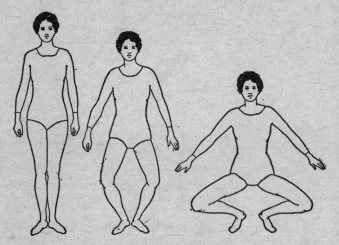

Borrowed from the classic ballet, this is a marvelous leg toner. Stand tall, with heels together (you may find it easier to balance yourself by holding on to the back of a chair with both hands). Keeping your back straight, begin bending your knees and slowly lower your body down to the floor. Lift your heels slightly. Slowly raise yourself to your starting position.

Leg Raises

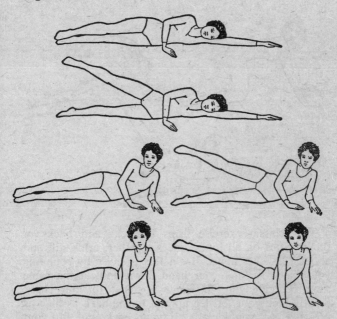

A super leg and inner-thigh trimmer. Lie flat on your side, right arm extended on the floor above your head. Support your body by placing left palm on the floor. Lift your leg high and lower it. Now raise your body a bit, supporting your weight on your right elbow. Kick your leg high. Last, raise your torso from the floor, supporting your weight wth both arms. Once more, kick up to the side. Repeat with other leg. (Note: don't overdo this one—do the side kicks stage by stage until you are comfortable with each level of difficulty.)

Donkey Kicks

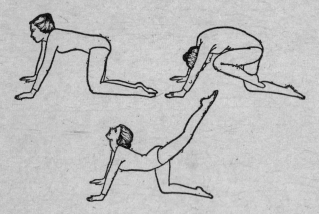

This classic exercise firms buttocks and backs of thighs. Start on all fours, knees together, arms stiff and about 12 inches apart. Begin this exercise by rounding your back, tucking your head down and, at the same time, bringing your left knee up close to your chest. Swiftly kick your left leg up and to the back as high as possible. As you kick, arch your back and lift your head. Lower your leg and repeat with right leg.

Knee-to-Chest Lifts

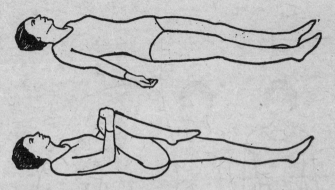

Stretch your thighs this way. Start on your back, arms at sides. Bend your right knee and lift it up close to your chest. Pull your knee to your chest by clasping your arms around it and pulling. Release and lower leg. Repeat with left leg.

Side Bends

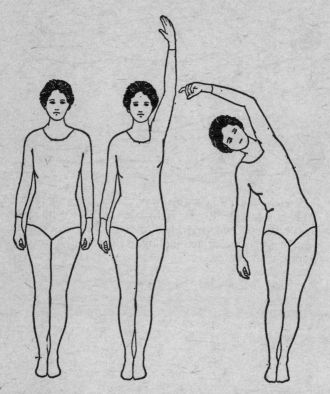

Shape your waist with this swinging routine. Stand with your legs close together, arms at sides. Raise your left arm above your head and bend sideways to the right—you should feel a slight pull in your left side. Bounce to the right a few times and return to starting position. Repeat exercise to the left side.

Little Jumps

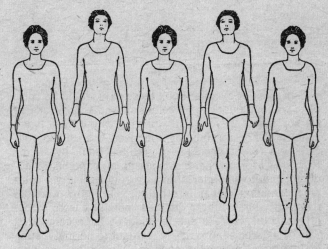

Finish your exercise program by jumping in place . . . a marvelous way to loosen your limbs and just plain relax. Little jumps are fine: keep your arms at your side or raise them to the side. This exercise is best done to lively music, where you can really let yourself go.

CELLULITE

What diet or exercise book these days would be complete without a note about cellulite? Apparently our European sisters have been worrying about this figure problem for years, but for American women the concern is a recent one. The bestselling book by Nicole Ronsard (Morrow, hardcover; Bantam, paperback) has done much to stir interest in this troublesome yet common condition. What is cellulite? The term describes those fatty lumps, those dimpled "cottage cheese" areas of the body where a special kind of fat accumulates. This "fat" seems inordinately resistant to normal dieting and exercise, hence the concern. Most often, cellulite accumulates on thighs, hips and buttocks, and if you have it, you know exactly what I'm talking about.

Theories as to the cause of cellulite are numerous, but the two popular ones lay the blame on chronic circulatory disorders of the connective tissue, or on the accumulation of waters and toxic materials in certain localized areas of the body. Research on the subject is not at all complete and certainly inconclusive at this time, but the problem remains an unsightly and embarrassing one for many, many women.

We are familiar, however, with several factors that provoke this condition: the stress of our modern life, shallow and ineffective breathing, fatigue, lack of exercise, overindulgence in drugs, alcohol and tobacco, poor posture and high estrogen levels in the female body. Genetic factors may also play a determining role.

Can one do anything about cellulite? Is it possible to get rid of those hard bumps beneath the skin and restore the smoothness of our younger years? Experts say yes.

What's called for are a number of specific actions, all of which must be followed faithfully for best results:

1. *A high-protein diet* is essential. You may follow any of the high-protein or low-carbohydrate diets in this book which allow fruits and vegetables, skim milk and milk products and very limited amounts of bread. It is imperative to drink 6–8 glasses of water each day. If you are overweight *and* are plagued with cellulite, it is natural to select one of these weight-loss regimes. If you are not overweight but have cellulite in one or several spots, simply add to the permitted quantities of food on the diet you choose, so that you will not be losing weight—only eating the right kinds of foods.

2. *Regular elimination* is crucial in order that toxic matters be removed from the body before they "poison" it. Proper elimination is possible with sensible eating habits, relaxation and a regular bathroom schedule. Do not get to depend on laxatives, which take up the normal functions of your own body.

3. *Relaxation* is difficult to achieve in this day and age. Do try to set aside at least an hour each day totally devoted to relaxation. Clear your mind of all worries, any disturbing thoughts—they'll wait for you. Think pleasant thoughts. Relaxation needn't be passive; you may find a rigorous game of tennis or an hour with an entertaining book the perfect looser-upper.

4. *Deep breathing* purifies the system by carrying large amounts of oxygen to every corner of the body. Whenever you think of it, but at least three times a day, perform the Deep Breathing Exercise described on page 174.

5. *Massage* may either be administered by a professional or be self-massage, which you can perform in your own home. Twenty minutes a day is recommended and, of course, you concentrate on the affected areas of the body. The traditional massage techniques are used: light stroking, pinching, kneading, knuckling and stroking all encourage circulation and develop muscle tone. If you are unfamiliar with massage technique, there are any number of inexpensive paperback books for the layperson which describe "how to do it."

Experts suggest that if your cellulite problem is especially severe, you should consult a physician for treatment. It is possible that hormonal imbalances may be causing an internal disturbance, but only a physician would be able to diagnose such a condition.

SUMMARY

Will you find a diet you can follow? Will you lose weight? And if you do, what are your chances of regaining once you've reduced? Unfortunately, not even the experts can predict a particular person's diet success or failure. All the studies into the nature of overweight and all the statistics in the world can't estimate how really serious you are about getting thin and staying thin. In the final analysis, it's your own desire to shed those pounds and keep them off—forever—that counts. The stronger your ambition and willpower, the greater your chances of success. If you really want to be thin, you will be.

I hope this book has fortified your initial determination to lose weight. I've guessed that you bought it for the obvious reason: you looked in the mirror and knew you needed to find a good diet. And, of course, that has been my primary goal: to provide you, the prospective dieter, with an ample selection of diets from which to choose a workable, effective program, the best one for you. I have included, as well as today's most talked-about diets, other weight-loss regimes that have retained their popularity over the years, diets I especially like because they show quick, dependable results.

With such a wide range of plans, you should have no trouble finding a diet you like. If it's a matter of five or so pounds that have started showing around your waist-line, they can be whisked away within a week on one of the crash diets described. Consult your palate, consider your stomach and then select a one-food crash that satisfies both. Whether it's strawberries, hot dogs or sparkling wine that makes you tingle, that crash—followed to the dot—will smooth away wrinkles and bulges faster than any other type of diet.

The low-carbohydrate diets are radical, and I recommend them if you've tried and failed on other diets before. On the one hand, they provide an abrupt shift in eating patterns, which is beneficial for some people; on the other, they limit carbohydrate intake to an absolute minimum, and carbohydrates, as you know, encourage excess pounds faster than any other food. The low-carb approach works well if (admit it!) you lack restraint when it comes to eating. Though you will eventually have to develop this trait if you are to stay slim, these plans allow you to learn at a more gentle pace. You can eat virtually unlimited amounts of protein and, on some plans, vegetables too, and still lose lots of weight. This, by the way, is another virtue: low-carbohydrate diets usually work super fast.

Low-calorie dieting is slower, steadier, and ultimately more reliable. "Cutting down" the portions on your plate and "cutting out" surplus calories guarantee a change in your figure; on most low-calorie diets you'll lose two to three pounds weekly. Not for the rambunctious or the incautious, calorie-counting plans are by nature conservative; you must stay within certain carefully proscribed food fences, eating only those items which your plan permits. Those who are blessed with a sturdy will and have a relatively easy time losing weight are the most likely candidates for low-calorie diets.

Personally, I think group action plans are marvelous. Their success ratios are impressive and they do provide what no other diets can: companionship, peer support and encouragement, a warm and friendly atmosphere, the information and advice of experts and the regularity imposed by scheduled weekly meetings. Consider Weight Watchers, TOPS, OA, or The Diet Workshop if you like to be with people and feel discouraged dieting alone. Group dieting has worked for thousands, and it may be a pleasant method for you.

It takes strength to lose weight, and I applaud you for making the effort. I don't think anyone but another overweight person realizes how impossible the task can seem, whether it's 10 pounds or 50 that have to go, so you deserve a resounding cheer for facing the problem head-on. Just keep reminding yourself as you struggle through the difficult days of your diet (and you'll have them, for sure) that you can do it. You, too, can be thin.

In addition to the diets themselves, I have included several chapters about the problem of "fat." I just can't stress enough how crucial it is for anyone going on a diet to read about the general problem of overweight. Knowing what fat is, why it "struck" you, how you can get it off, what fat does to your body and your health and which foods are fat-promoting, is absolutely essential. Ignoring this part of the problem is like trying to fix the engine of a car without knowing how an automobile works. In the long run, the cure won't work; the car will break down again. Diets are often just stop-gap, temporary measures, too. They are not, in themselves, cures for fat, though they can be. If we simply jump, like overfed sheep, onto the bandwagon of every new diet craze that appears, we'll never succeed in staying thin once and for all. Understanding why we are overweight is the only way to solve the problem permanently.

As I've noted in earlier chapters, there's no one scapegoat for fat, no single reason why millions of Americans are overweight. The problem is more complex, the aggravating factors cumulative. Our high standard of living, our designation of food as security and status, the advent of processed snack foods and their "freezability," our sedentary life-styles and the mushrooming of fast-food eateries are just a few reasons. The psychological importance we've attached to our food accounts for millions more pounds; food represents love, warmth, home and safety in an America that is undergoing enormous social upheavals and massive change. Food is the constant we've learned to rely on for security. All these elements are making us bulge and strain at our American seams.

This national problem does have its positive side, however, a sort of silver lining in the plump rain cloud. Research into obesity has increased tremendously over the past decades, and what we've learned has filled volumes and libraries. A new field of scientific inquiry has been spawned, and what we're learning is that obesity is a disease, much like other diseases.

Medically, there's been progress. We know now that obesity sometimes has its genesis in distinct physiological conditions, identifiable malfunctions of the body's various systems: the endocrine glands, the metabolic processes, the blood sugar. Being able to pinpoint these causative factors has led to a swift reversal of obesity in conditions that were once considered incurable. People who could never lose weight before are finally able to reduce, only because research has made the link between our body chemistry and fat. On the other hand, obesity has been named as a contributing cause to certain other medical conditions: heart disease, diabetes, kidney dysfunction and gall bladder disease, among others. Being able to control an individual's weight has improved immeasurably the health and lives of patients suffering from these related diseases.

What else have we learned? For one thing, scientific research has exploded the myth of "miracle diet pills," the amphetamine drugs so widely used in the treatment of overweight up until very recently. Dieters are now warned against the indiscriminate use of appetite suppressants for dieting purposes. As well as producing undesirable side-effects such as insomnia, anxiety, general nervousness, high blood pressure, rapid heartbeat and gastrointestinal disturbances, which some "pep pills" do, these drugs induce a state of psychological dependence. Medical researchers have observed hundreds of cases of addiction to these drugs, notoriously among suburban women to whom they were commonly dispensed by doctors for weight control.

Psychological research into the problems of the obese is relatively recent, also. No longer considered the "jolly fat woman" or man, the overweight individual is taken seriously in psychological circles, and acceptance made of the fact that obesity often evidences deeper psychological disturbances. Some professionals even specialize in the treatment of the obese. Which is not to say that *you* specifically have severe mental problems just because you're overweight; only that *some* people who are fat are also terribly unhappy. Various types of therapy are now widely available for these persons, and there should be no shame in seeking individual therapy, group therapy or counseling or a course in behavior modification, which is a retraining technique adapted to help overweights change harmful eating patterns.

Nutrition has received serious attention in this postwar era, at least in part as a direct result of our national fat problem. We're overweight, reasoned the experts, and that fact must have something to do with what we're eating! Experts know more today about the nature and composition of foods than ever before. They can distinguish the particular traits of various nutrients—proteins, carbohydrates, fats—and foretell their effects on the body. They have also explored the little-researched subject of vitamins and are now investigating vitamin therapy as an adjunctive nutrition field. And because experts know more, we, too, are more aware than ever before about how the food we eat affects us. Armed with facts, we are able to choose diets that provide for our best health and well-being.

The food industry has also come under closer scrutiny. Increased supervision and monitoring of food processing and packaging are prevalent, and the newly passed food labeling laws, which inform the public about the nutritional content of our foods, are a long-awaited step in a positive direction.

Perhaps the most important development to come with the fuss about overweight and diet is a growing interest in and concern with health. Our health and our children's. As well as realizing the need to control weight for the sake of attractiveness, we are fast concluding that a slim figure, a nutritionally balanced diet, and a life that includes work and play, restful and active pursuits, best promotes the health and well-being of all of us. Exercise in the form of sports—jogging, tennis, skiing, long-distance running—continues to draw growing numbers of enthusiasts each year. We are finally realizing that regular physical activity, which firms muscles and makes our hearts strong and resilient, is one of the very best ways to ensure overall health. Fortunately, the interest doesn't seem to be faddish.

On the diet front, there are more new interesting diets all the time to aid us overweights in reducing. As our knowledge of medicine, nutrition and health increases, diets become more sophisticated and precise, hence, more effective. As we, the public, become better acquainted in these areas and begin to assume responsibility for our own health, we are developing the confidence to create our own diet plans, based on our individual body needs and personal life-styles.

I'll close with this thought: it takes courage to lose weight. It takes greater courage to keep weight off. While sticking with your diet is important (and you *will* stick with it, won't you?), modifying eating patterns is perhaps the most crucial part of any diet. We must all be aware of the reasons—different, indeed, in every case—why we are fat. We must resolve to change our habits once and forever.

Being thin is easy—once you really want to.

Good luck.

FOOD AND
BEVERAGE COUNTER

Are strawberries higher in carbohydrates than blue-berries? Is there more fat in a pork chop than in a lamb chop? Is a glass of tomato juice higher in calories than a glass of grapefruit juice? Does a cup of cottage cheese contain more protein than a cup of yogurt?

You'll find the answers to these questions (and many, many more) in the counter that follows. Listed alphabetically, the counter gives the calorie, protein, fat and carbohydrate gram content of over 1500 foods and beverages.

Food values. For those who are counting calories or carbohydrates, the counter will prove invaluable for menu planning and for determining your daily food allowances. The protein content will be helpful to those who want to diet the high-protein way, and the fat content listing will benefit dieters who are also watching their intake of fat.

Food weights and measures. Whenever possible, the foods are given in common household measures (i.e., 1 cup, 4 ounces, 1 pound, 1 tablespoon, etc.), but if you want to be truly accurate, pay close attention to the gram weight listed. It's not there just for metric conversion; it's there to tell you *exactly* how much something weighs, since food values are all based upon that specified weight.

Knowing the gram weight will prove especially helpful in determining foods listed by size. If, for example, you want to eat an orange, you'll find a Florida orange listed the following way: " . . . . . 1 average (3″ diameter) . . . . . " This doesn't mean you should take a tapemeasure to the supermarket. But if you want to be precise, just buy an inexpensive gram scale, and weigh the orange (or anything else in question) to see how its weight compares with the weight specified here. In this case, an "average" Florida orange weighs 210 grams. If your orange weighs only 190 grams, it's approximately 10% smaller. You can then adjust all the food values by 10%, and eat your orange.

Knowing the gram weight also helps in checking out foods listed by measure. If, for example, your cup of cooked green beans weighs more than the figure listed here (which is 130 grams), it's probably packed tighter than "average." The gram weight will quickly tell you, so that you can make the necessary adjustment (in either the beans or the food values).

Bear in mind that all portions listed pertain only to the *edible part of the food*. If you're drinking a glass of milk, this doesn't matter since milk is all edible. But it does matter if you're eating a food such as watermelon. An entire wedge of watermelon may weigh about 2 pounds, and the gram weight will indicate this. However, the food value data applies only to the part of melon that's edible—which is approximately 25% of the entire wedge.

Origin of food values. Every figure in this book was compiled on the basis of data available from the United States Department of Agriculture. As noted above, the food values are all based on the edible portions of foods listed.

Abbreviations

n.a.	not available
oz.	ounce
lb.	pound

Food and measure	gram weight	calories	protein grams	fat grams	carbo-hydrate grams
Abalone, canned, 4 oz.	114	91	18.1	.3	2.6
Abalone, raw, 4 oz.	114	111	21.2	.6	3.8
Acerola juice, 6 oz. glass	188	43	.8	.6	9.0
Alcoholic beverages:					
beer, 4.5% alcohol, 12 oz. glass	360	151	n.a.	n.a.	13.7
pure distilled gin, rum, whiskey, vodka, etc.:					
80 proof, 1½ oz. jigger	42	97	n.a.	n.a.	trace
86 proof, 1½ oz. jigger	42	104	n.a.	n.a.	trace
90 proof, 1½ oz. jigger	42	110	n.a.	n.a.	trace
94 proof, 1½ oz. jigger	42	115	n.a.	n.a.	trace
100 proof, 1½ oz. jigger	42	124	n.a.	n.a.	trace
wine, dessert, 18.8% alcohol, 3½ oz. glass ..	103	141	.1	0	7.9
wine, table, 12.2% alcohol, 3½ oz. glass	102	87	.1	0	4.3
Alewife, canned with liquid, 4 oz.	114	161	18.5	9.1	0
Almonds:					
dried, in shell, 4 oz.	114	346	10.8	31.4	11.3
dried, shelled, 4 oz.	114	678	21.1	61.5	22.1
dried, shelled, ½ cup	71	425	13.2	38.5	13.8
roasted, shelled, 4 oz.	114	711	21.1	65.4	22.1
roasted, shelled, ½ cup	78	489	14.5	45.0	15.2

Food and measure	gram weight	calories	protein grams	fat grams	carbohydrate grams
chopped, ½ cup ··············	64	401	11.9	36.9	12.5
candy and chocolate coated, see *Candies* .					
Anchovies, canned in oil, 1 oz. ·········	28	50	5.4	2.9	trace
Anchovy paste, 1 tablespoon ··········	20	42	1.6	2.0	.9
Apple butter, 1 tablespoon ··········	15	28	trace	.1	7.0
Apple juice, canned, 6 oz. glass ·········	187	91	.2	trace	22.2
Apples:					
raw, average commercial variety, whole, 1 lb.	454	242	.8	2.5	60.5
raw, unpared, 1 average (about 3 per lb.) ..	150	80	.3	.8	20.0
raw, pared, diced, 1 cup ·········	109	59	.2	.3	15.4
raw, pared, quartered, 1 cup ········	122	66	.2	.4	17.2
dehydrated, uncooked, 4 oz. ·······	114	400	1.6	2.3	104.4
dehydrated rings, uncooked, 1 cup ········	86	304	1.2	1.7	79.2
dried, cooked, sweetened, 1 cup ·········	280	314	.8	1.0	81.5
dried, cooked, unsweetened, 1 cup ········	260	202	.8	1.2	52.5
frozen, sweetened, 4 oz. ··········	114	105	.2	.1	27.5
frozen slices, sweetened, 1 cup ·········	200	186	.4	.2	48.6
Applesauce, canned, sweetened, 1 cup ·······	255	232	.5	.3	60.7
Applesauce, canned, unsweetened, 1 cup ······	244	100	.5	.5	26.3
Apricot nectar, canned, 6 oz. glass ········	188	107	.6	.2	27.4

	Grams	Calories	Protein	Fat	Carbohydrate
Apricots:					
raw, whole, 1 lb.	454	217	4.3	.9	54.6
raw, 1 average (about 12 per lb.)	38	18	.4	trace	4.5
raw, pitted, halved, 1 cup	156	80	1.6	.3	19.9
canned in heavy syrup, 1 cup	252	217	1.5	.2	55.4
canned in heavy syrup, drained, 1 cup	217	186	1.3	.2	47.7
dried, uncooked, 4 oz.	114	295	5.7	.6	75.4
dried, uncooked, 1 cup	150	390	7.5	.7	99.7
dried, cooked, sweetened, 1 cup	325	396	4.6	.3	102.2
dried, cooked, unsweetened, 1 cup	285	242	4.6	.6	61.6
frozen, sweetened, 1 cup	260	256	1.8	.2	65.2
candied, 1 oz.	28	96	.1	trace	24.5
Artichoke hearts, frozen, 3 average	85	22	1.2	.2	4.9
Artichokes, French, boiled, 1 average	120	53	3.3	.3	11.9
Asparagus:					
raw spears, 1 lb.	454	66	6.4	.5	12.7
fresh, cooked, drained, 4 spears	60	12	1.3	.1	2.2
fresh cuts, cooked, drained, 1 cup	145	29	3.2	.3	5.2
canned spears, drained, 1 cup	215	45	5.2	.9	7.3
frozen spears, 4 oz.	114	27	3.6	.2	4.4
frozen cuts and tips, 1 cup	180	41	5.9	.4	6.5
Avacados, fresh:					
California, peeled and pitted, ½ average	108	185	2.4	18.3	6.5

Food and measure	gram weight	calories	protein grams	fat grams	carbo-hydrate grams
Florida, peeled and pitted, ½ average	123	157	1.6	13.5	10.8
diced, 1 cup	147	245	3.1	24.1	9.3
mashed, 1 cup	231	386	4.8	37.9	14.5
Bacon, Canadian, cooked crisp, drained, 1 slice	15	42	4.1	2.6	trace
Bacon, cooked crisp, drained, 2 slices	15	92	4.5	7.8	.5
Bagel, egg, 1 medium (3" diameter)	55	165	6.0	2.0	28.0
Bagel, water, 1 medium (3" diameter)	55	165	6.0	2.0	30.0
Baking powder, dry:					
phosphate, 2 tablespoons	27	33	trace	trace	7.9
SAS-phosphate, 2 tablespoons	22	28	trace	trace	5.5
tartrate, 2 tablespoons	23	18	trace	trace	4.3
Bamboo shoots, fresh, 4 oz.	114	31	2.9	.3	5.9
Bananas: fresh, whole, 1 lb.	454	262	3.4	.6	68.5
peeled, 1 medium	119	101	1.3	.2	26.4
sliced, 1 cup	146	124	1.6	.3	32.4
mashed, 1 cup	222	189	2.4	.4	49.3
baking type, plantain, peeled, 1 medium	126	150	1.4	.5	39.3
dehydrated flakes, 1 cup	100	340	4.4	.8	88.6
Barbecue sauce, 1 cup	250	228	3.7	17.2	20.0

	Grams	Calories	Protein	Fat	Carbohydrate
Barley, pearled, light, uncooked, 1 cup	200	698	16.4	2.0	157.6
Barley, pearled, pot or Scotch, uncooked, 1 cup	200	696	19.2	2.2	154.4
Bass, sea, raw, 4 oz.	114	116	21.9	1.4	0
Bass, striped, raw, 4 oz.	114	120	21.5	3.1	0
Bean sprouts, mung, raw, 1 cup	90	32	3.4	.2	6.0
Bean sprouts, soy, raw, 1 cup	107	49	6.6	1.5	5.7
Beans, baked, canned:					
in tomato sauce, 8 oz.	227	272	14.3	1.1	52.2
with frankfurters, 8 oz.	227	327	17.3	16.1	28.6
with pork in tomato sauce, 8 oz.	227	277	13.8	5.9	43.1
with pork in molasses sauce, 8 oz.	227	340	14.0	10.7	47.8
Beans, green or snap:					
raw, whole, 1 lb.	454	128	7.6	.8	28.3
raw, cuts, 1 cup	105	34	2.0	.2	7.5
fresh, cooked, drained, cuts, 1 cup	130	33	2.1	.3	7.0
canned, cuts, drained, 1 cup	140	34	2.0	.3	7.3
canned, cuts, with liquid, 1 cup	230	42	2.4	.2	9.6
frozen, cuts, boiled, drained, 1 cup	160	40	2.5	.2	9.1
Beans, lima:					
raw, immature, in pods, 1 lb.	454	223	15.2	.9	40.1
fresh, boiled, drained, 1 cup	170	189	12.9	.9	33.7
canned, drained, 1 cup	175	168	9.5	.5	32.0
frozen, baby, boiled, drained, 1 cup	173	204	12.8	.3	38.6

Food and measure	gram weight	calories	protein grams	fat grams	carbo-hydrate grams
frozen, fordhook, boiled, drained, 1 cup · · · ·	168	166	10.1	.2	32.1
Beans, red kidney:					
dry, 1 cup ·	186	638	41.8	2.8	115.1
cooked, drained, 1 cup · · · · · · · · · · · · · · ·	185	218	14.4	.9	39.6
canned, with liquid, 1 cup · · · · · · · · · · · ·	256	230	14.6	1.0	41.9
Beans, pinto, calico, Mexican, dry, 4 oz. · · · ·	114	396	26.1	1.4	72.6
Beans, wax, boiled, drained, 1 cup · · · · · · · · ·	140	31	2.0	.3	6.4
Beans, wax, canned, drained, 1 cup · · · · · · · ·	140	34	1.6	.4	7.3
Beans, white, dry, 1 cup · · · · · · · · · · · · · · ·	200	680	44.6	3.2	122.6
Beans, white, boiled, drained, 1 cup · · · · · · ·	190	224	14.8	1.1	40.3
Beechnuts, in shell, 4 oz. · · · · · · · · · · · · · ·	114	393	13.4	34.6	14.1
Beechnuts, shelled, 4 oz. · · · · · · · · · · · · · · ·	114	644	22.0	56.7	23.0
Beef, choice grade, retail trim, meat only, 4 oz.:					
chuck, boneless arm, pot roasted, lean and fat	114	329	30.9	21.8	0
chuck, boneless arm, pot roasted, lean only · ·	114	220	34.7	7.9	0
club steak, broiled, lean and fat · · · · · · · · · ·	114	517	23.5	46.3	0
club steak, broiled, lean only · · · · · · · · · · · ·	114	278	33.7	14.8	0
flank steak, pot roasted · · · · · · · · · · · · · · · ·	114	223	34.8	8.3	0
ground, lean, raw ·	114	203	23.5	11.3	0
ground, lean, broiled · · · · · · · · · · · · · · · · · ·	114	250	31.2	12.9	0

ground, regular, broiled	114	326	27.6	23.1	0
porterhouse steak, broiled, lean and fat	114	530	22.4	48.1	0
porterhouse steak, broiled, lean only	114	255	34.4	11.9	0
rib, roasted, lean and fat	114	502	22.7	44.9	0
rib, roasted, lean only	114	275	32.1	15.2	0
round, broiled, lean and fat	114	297	32.6	17.5	0
round, broiled, lean only	114	214	35.5	6.9	0
rump, roasted, lean and fat	114	395	26.9	31.1	0
rump, roasted, lean only	114	237	33.1	10.6	0
sirloin steak, double-bone, broiled, lean and fat	114	465	25.3	39.5	0
sirloin steak, double-bone, broiled, lean only	114	246	34.8	10.8	0
sirloin steak, round-bone, broiled, lean and fat	114	441	26.2	36.5	0
sirloin steak, round-bone, broiled, lean only	114	236	36.7	8.7	0
T-bone steak, broiled, lean and fat	114	539	22.2	49.2	0
T-bone steak, broiled, lean only	114	254	34.6	11.7	0
Beef, corned:					
boiled, medium fat, 4 oz.	114	424	26.1	34.6	0
canned, fat, 4 oz.	114	298	26.6	20.4	0
canned, medium fat, 4 oz.	114	245	28.7	13.6	0
canned, lean, 4 oz.	114	210	29.9	9.1	0
canned, hash, with potato, 1 cup	220	398	19.4	24.9	23.5
Beef, dried or chipped uncooked, 4 oz.	114	231	39.1	6.2	0

Food and measure	gram weight	calories	protein grams	fat grams	carbo-hydrate grams
Beef, potted, 4 oz.	114	283	19.9	21.9	0
Beef, roast, canned, 4 oz.	114	254	28.3	14.8	0
Beef liver, see *Liver*					
Beef pot pie, frozen, 8 oz. pie	227	436	16.6	22.5	40.9
Beef stew, with vegetables, canned, 8 oz.	227	179	13.2	7.0	16.1
Beef tongue, see *Tongue*					
Beer, see *Alcoholic Beverages*					
Beet greens, raw, 1 lb.	454	61	5.6	.8	11.7
Beet greens, boiled, drained, 1 cup	200	36	3.4	.4	6.6
Beets:					
raw, trimmed, 1 lb.	454	137	5.1	.3	31.4
raw, 1 medium (2″ diameter)	50	21	.8	trace	4.9
fresh, diced, boiled, drained, 1 cup	180	58	2.0	.2	12.9
fresh, sliced, boiled, drained, 1 cup	205	66	2.2	.2	14.8
canned, diced, drained, 1 cup	163	60	1.6	.2	14.3
canned, sliced, drained, 1 cup	176	65	1.8	.2	15.5
canned, whole, drained, 1 cup	159	59	1.6	.2	14.0
Beverages, see individual listings					
Biscuit dough, canned, chilled, 4 oz.	114	318	8.3	7.3	52.9
Biscuit dough, canned, frozen, 4 oz.	114	263	6.5	13.6	55.7

Food					
Biscuit mix, baked with milk, 1 oz. biscuit	28	92	2.0	2.6	14.8
Blackberries:					
fresh, 1 lb.	454	250	5.2	3.9	55.6
fresh, washed, 1 cup	146	85	1.8	1.3	18.8
canned, with heavy syrup, 1 cup	260	237	2.1	1.6	57.7
frozen, sweetened, 1 cup	252	242	2.0	.8	61.5
Blackberry juice, canned, 6 oz. glass	184	68	.6	1.1	14.4
Blackeye peas, see Cowpeas					
Blueberries:					
fresh, 1 lb.	454	259	2.9	2.1	63.8
fresh, 1 cup	146	90	1.2	.4	35.6
canned, with syrup, 1 cup	250	253	1.0	.5	65.0
frozen, sweetened, 1 cup	228	239	1.4	.7	60.4
frozen, unsweetened, 1 cup	165	91	1.2	.8	22.4
Bluefish, baked or broiled with butter, 4 oz.	114	181	29.9	5.9	0
Bockwurst, 4 oz.	114	301	12.9	27.0	.7
Bologna, all meat, 4 oz.	114	312	14.9	25.6	4.2
Bologna, with cereal added, 4 oz.	114	299	16.2	23.5	4.4
Bouillon cube, ½" cube	4	5	.8	.1	.2
Brains, all kinds, raw, 4 oz.	114	142	11.8	9.8	.9
Boysenberries, see Blackberries					
Braunschweiger, 4 oz.	114	364	16.9	31.2	2.6
Brazil nuts:					

Food and measure	gram weight	calories	protein grams	fat grams	carbohydrate grams
in shell, 4 oz.	114	356	7.8	36.4	5.9
shelled, 4 oz.	114	741	16.2	75.9	12.4
shelled, 1 cup	142	929	20.3	95.0	15.5
shelled, 2–3 nuts	10	65	1.4	6.7	1.1
Bread:					
Boston brown, 1 slice, 3 × ¾"	48	101	2.6	.6	21.9
cracked wheat, 1 lb. loaf	454	1193	39.5	10.0	236.3
cracked wheat, 1 slice (20 per loaf) ...	23	60	2.0	.5	11.9
French or Vienna, 1 lb. loaf	454	1316	41.3	13.6	251.5
French or Vienna, 1 slice, 3¼ × 2 × 1" ..	20	58	1.8	.6	11.1
Italian, 1 lb. loaf	454	1253	41.3	3.6	256.0
Italian, 1 slice, 3¼ × 2 × 1"	20	55	1.8	.1	11.3
pumpernickel, 1 lb. loaf	454	1117	41.3	5.4	241.1
pumpernickel, 1 slice, 3¾ × 3¾ × ⅛" ...	30	74	2.7	.4	15.9
raisin, 1 lb. loaf	454	1189	29.9	12.7	243.3
raisin, 1 slice (20 per loaf)	23	60	1.5	.6	12.3
rye, light, 1 lb. loaf	454	1103	41.3	5.0	236.5
rye, light, 1 slice (20 per loaf)	23	56	2.1	.2	11.9
rye, light, 1 party slice, 3 × 2 × ½" ..	15	36	1.3	.1	7.8
white, 1 lb. loaf	454	1225	39.5	14.5	229.3

white, 1 slice (20 per loaf)	23	62	2.0	.7	11.6
white, 1 thin slice (26 per loaf)	17	46	1.5	.5	8.6
whole wheat, 1 lb. loaf	454	1103	47.7	13.6	216.5
whole wheat, 1 slice (20 per loaf)	23	56	2.4	.7	11.0
Breadcrumbs, dry, grated, 1 oz.	28	111	3.6	1.3	20.8
Breadcrumbs, dry, grated, 1 cup	102	400	12.9	4.7	74.9
Breadfruit, peeled and trimmed, 4 oz.	114	117	1.9	.3	29.9
Breadfruit, raw, untrimmed, 1 lb.	454	360	5.9	1.0	91.5
Bread sticks, regular, 1 oz.	28	109	3.4	.8	21.3
Bread sticks, Vienna, 1 oz.	28	86	2.7	.9	16.4
Bread stuffing mix, dry, 4 oz.	114	421	14.6	4.3	82.1
Bread stuffing mix, dry, 1 cup	71	263	9.1	2.7	51.4
Broccoli:					
raw, trimmed spears, 1 lb.	454	89	10.0	.8	16.3
fresh, spears, boiled, drained, 1 cup	150	39	4.6	.4	6.7
fresh, cuts, boiled, drained, 1 cup	155	40	4.8	.5	7.0
frozen, spears, 10 oz. package	283	79	9.3	.6	14.4
frozen, chopped, boiled, drained, 1 cup	188	49	5.5	.6	8.6
Brussels sprouts:					
raw, trimmed, 1 lb.	454	188	20.4	1.7	34.6
fresh, boiled, drained, 1 cup	180	65	7.6	.7	11.5
frozen, boiled, drained, 1 cup	188	62	6.0	.4	12.2
Buckwheat, see *Flour*					

Food and measure	gram weight	calories	protein grams	fat grams	carbohydrate grams
Bulgar, parboiled wheat:					
club, dry, 4 oz.	114	407	9.7	1.6	90.2
hard red winter, dry, 4 oz.	114	401	12.7	1.7	85.8
white, dry, 4 oz.	114	405	11.7	1.4	88.6
canned, hard red winter, seasoned, 1 cup	135	246	8.4	4.5	44.3
canned, hard red winter, seasoned, 4 oz.	114	206	8.3	3.7	37.2
canned, hard red winter, unseasoned, 4 oz.	114	191	8.3	.8	39.7
Butter:					
1 cup or ½ lb.	227	1625	1.4	183.9	.9
1 tablespoon	14	100	.1	11.3	trace
1 pat, 1 × ⅓" (90 per lb.)	5	36	trace	4.0	trace
whipped, 8 oz. container	227	1625	1.4	183.9	.9
whipped, 1 stick or ½ cup	76	544	.5	61.5	.3
whipped, 1 tablespoon	9	64	.1	7.3	trace
Buttermilk, see *Milk*					
Butternuts, in shell, 4 oz.	114	100	3.8	9.7	1.3
Butternuts, shelled, 4 oz.	114	713	26.9	69.4	9.5
Butternuts, 4-5 nuts	15	94	3.5	9.2	1.3
Butter oil, 1 tablespoon	14	123	trace	13.9	0

Cabbage:

common, raw, trimmed, 1 lb.	454	98	5.3	.8	22.0
common, raw, chopped, 1 cup	89	21	1.2	.2	4.8
common, raw, coarse shredded, 1 cup	70	22	.9	.1	3.8
common, shredded, boiled, drained, 1 cup	145	29	1.6	.3	6.2
common, wedges, boiled, drained, 1 cup	184	33	1.8	.4	7.4
common, raw, salad, see Coleslaw					
red, raw, trimmed, 1 lb.	454	127	8.2	.8	28.2
red, raw, chopped, 1 cup	89	28	1.8	.2	6.1
red, raw, coarse shredded, 1 cup	70	22	1.4	.1	4.8
savoy, raw, trimmed, 1 lb.	454	98	9.8	.8	18.8
savoy, raw, coarse shredded, 1 cup	70	17	1.7	.1	3.2
Cabbage, Chinese, raw, 1 lb.	454	62	5.3	.4	13.2
Cabbage, Chinese, raw, 1" cuts, 1 cup	75	11	.9	.1	2.2
Cabbage, Chinese, raw, strips, 1 cup	59	8	.7	.1	1.8
Cabbage, spoon, raw, 1 lb.	454	69	6.9	.9	12.5
Cabbage, spoon, boiled, drained, 1 cup	170	24	2.4	.3	4.1
Cake, devil's food, frozen, with icing, 4 oz.	114	433	4.9	20.1	63.4
Cake icing, see Icing					
Cake mixes, dry form and prepared; 4 oz.:					
angel food, dry form	114	439	9.6	11.6	100.9
angel food, prepared with water, flavoring	114	295	6.5	.2	67.7
chocolate malt, dry form	114	470	4.6	12.2	90.1

Food and measure	gram weight	calories	protein grams	fat grams	carbo-hydrate grams
chocolate malt, prep. with eggs, water, icing ..	114	394	3.9	9.9	75.9
coffeecake, dry form	114	491	6.7	12.5	88.0
coffeecake, prep. with eggs, milk	114	367	7.2	10.9	59.7
devil's food, dry form	114	463	5.5	13.3	87.8
devil's food, prep. with eggs, water, icing ..	114	386	5.0	14.0	66.5
gingerbread, dry form	114	485	6.2	11.9	89.1
gingerbread, prep. with water	114	315	3.5	7.8	58.2
honey spice, dry form	114	505	4.9	16.0	87.0
honey spice, prep with eggs, water, icing	114	401	4.8	12.3	69.4
marble, dry form	114	485	5.6	15.4	86.2
marble, prep. with eggs, water, icing	114	377	5.0	9.9	70.7
white, dry form	114	495	4.7	13.6	89.4
white, prep. with egg whites, water, icing ..	114	400	4.4	12.2	71.6
yellow, dry form	114	499	4.6	14.7	88.5
yellow, prep. with eggs, water, icing	114	384	4.7	12.9	65.7
Calves' liver, see *Liver*					
Candied fruit, see individual listings					
Candies, 1 oz.:					
almonds, chocolate coated	28	161	3.5	12.4	11.2
almonds, sugar coated	28	129	2.2	5.3	19.9

butterscotch	28	112	trace	1.0	26.9
candy corn	28	103	trace	.6	25.4
caramel, plain or chocolate	28	113	1.1	2.9	21.7
caramel, plain or chocolate, with nuts	28	121	1.3	4.6	20.0
caramel, chocolate flavored roll	28	112	.6	2.3	23.4
chocolate, bittersweet	28	135	2.2	11.2	13.2
chocolate, milk	28	147	2.2	9.2	16.1
chocolate, milk, with almonds	28	151	2.6	10.1	14.5
chocolate, milk, with peanuts	28	154	4.0	10.8	12.6
chocolate, milk, sugar coated	28	132	1.5	5.6	20.6
chocolate, semi-sweet	28	144	1.2	10.1	16.2
chocolate, sweet	28	147	1.2	9.9	16.4
chocolate fudge, chocolate coated	28	122	1.1	4.5	20.7
chocolate fudge with nuts, chocolate coated	28	128	1.4	5.9	19.0
coconut, chocolate coated	28	124	.8	5.0	20.4
fondant	28	103	trace	.6	25.4
fondant, chocolate coated	28	116	.5	3.0	23.0
fudge, chocolate	28	113	.8	3.5	21.3
fudge, chocolate, with nuts	28	121	1.1	4.9	19.6
fudge, vanilla	28	113	.9	3.1	21.2
fudge, vanilla, with nuts	28	120	1.2	4.6	19.5
fudge, with caramel, nuts, chocolate coated	28	123	2.2	5.1	18.2
fudge, with nuts, caramel, chocolate coated	28	130	2.7	6.5	16.6

Food and measure	gram weight	calories	protein grams	fat grams	carbohydrate grams
gum drops	28	98	trace	.2	24.8
hard candy	28	109	0	.3	27.6
honey with peanut butter, chocolate coated	28	131	1.9	5.5	20.0
jelly beans	28	104	trace	.1	26.4
marshmallows	28	90	.6	trace	22.8
mints, uncoated	28	103	trace	.6	25.4
nougat and caramel, chocolate coated	28	118	1.1	3.9	20.6
peanut bar	28	146	5.0	9.1	13.4
peanut brittle	28	119	1.6	2.9	23.0
peanuts, chocolate coated	28	159	4.6	11.7	11.1
raisins, chocolate coated	28	120	1.5	4.8	20.0
vanilla creams, chocolate coated	28	123	1.1	4.8	19.9
Cantaloupe, ½ melon (5" diameter)	385	58	1.4	.2	14.5
Cantaloupe, cubed, 1 cup	162	49	1.1	.2	12.2
Capicola, 4 oz.	114	565	22.9	51.9	0
Carrots:					
raw, without tops, 1 lb.	454	156	4.1	.7	36.1
raw, 1 medium (5½ × 1")	50	21	.5	.1	4.8
raw, chunks, 1 cup	138	58	1.5	.3	13.4
raw, diced, 1 cup	144	60	1.6	.3	14.0

raw, grated or shredded, 1 cup	109	46	1.2	.2	10.6
raw, slices, 1 cup	127	53	1.4	.3	12.3
raw, strips, 1 cup	117	49	1.3	.2	11.3
boiled, drained, chunks, 1 cup	164	51	1.5	.3	11.6
boiled, drained, diced, 1 cup	140	43	1.3	.3	9.9
boiled, drained, slices, 1 cup	153	47	1.4	.3	10.9
canned, diced, drained, 1 cup	159	48	1.3	.5	10.6
dehydrated, 1 oz.	28	97	1.9	.4	23.0
Casaba melon, flesh only, 4 oz.	114	31	1.4	trace	7.4
Casaba melon, cubed, 1 cup	162	44	1.9	trace	10.5
Cashew nuts, roasted, shelled, 4 oz.	114	639	19.6	52.1	33.4
Cashew nuts, roasted, shelled, 1 cup	140	785	24.1	64.0	41.0
Catsup, tomato, bottled, 1 cup	282	299	5.6	1.1	71.6
Catsup, tomato, bottled, 1 tablespoon	17	18	.3	trace	4.3
Cauliflower:					
raw, untrimmed, 1 lb.	454	48	4.8	.4	9.2
raw, flowerets only, 1 lb.	454	122	12.2	.9	23.6
raw, sliced, 1 cup	83	22	2.2	.2	4.3
boiled, drained, 1 cup	125	28	2.9	.3	5.1
frozen, boiled, drained, 1 cup	179	32	3.4	.4	5.9
Caviar, sturgeon, granular, 1 oz.	28	74	7.6	4.2	1.0
Caviar, sturgeon, pressed, 1 oz.	28	89	9.7	4.7	1.3
Celeriac root, raw, whole, 1 lb.	454	156	7.0	1.2	33.2

Food and measure	gram weight	calories	protein grams	fat grams	carbohydrate grams
Celeriac root, raw, pared, 4 oz.	114	45	2.0	.3	9.6
Celeriac root, raw, pared, 4–6 roots	100	40	1.8	.3	8.5
Celery:					
raw, untrimmed, 1 lb.	454	58	3.1	.3	13.3
raw, 1 outer stalk (8" long)	40	7	.4	trace	1.6
raw, chopped or finely diced, 1 cup	119	20	1.1	.1	4.6
raw, diced, or chunks, 1 cup	121	21	1.1	.1	4.7
raw, slices, 1 cup	106	18	1.0	.1	4.1
boiled, drained, diced or chunks, 1 cup ...	153	21	1.2	.2	4.7
boiled, drained, slices, 1 cup	168	24	1.3	.2	5.2
Celery cabbage, see *Cabbage, Chinese*					
Cereal, cooking-type, ¼ cup uncooked:					
farina, enriched	40	148	4.6	.4	30.8
farina, instant	40	145	4.6	.4	30.1
farina, quick cooking	40	145	4.6	.4	30.1
oats, with wheat germ, soy grits	20	76	4.1	1.8	11.7
oatmeal	20	78	2.8	1.5	13.6
wheat, rolled	25	85	2.5	.5	19.1
Cereal, ready-to-eat, 1 oz.:					
bran, with sugar, malt extract	28	68	3.6	.9	21.1

	28				
bran, with sugar, defatted wheat germ	28	67	3.1	.5	22.3
bran flakes, 40%	28	86	2.9	.5	22.8
bran flakes, with raisins	28	81	2.3	.4	22.5
corn, puffed	28	113	2.3	1.2	22.9
corn, puffed, presweetened	28	107	1.1	trace	25.4
corn, puffed, presweetened, cocoa flavor	28	110	1.7	.6	24.6
corn, puffed, presweetened, fruit flavor	28	112	1.6	.8	24.8
corn, shredded	28	110	2.0	.1	24.6
corn flakes	28	109	2.2	.1	24.2
corn flakes, sugar coated	28	109	1.2	trace	25.9
corn flakes, with protein concentrates	28	107	6.5	.5	19.0
corn, rice and wheat flakes	28	110	2.1	.2	24.4
oat flakes, with soy flour and rice	28	113	4.2	1.6	20.0
oats, puffed	28	113	3.4	1.6	21.3
oats, puffed, sugar coated	28	112	1.9	1.0	24.3
oats, shredded	28	107	5.3	.6	20.4
rice, puffed	28	113	1.7	.1	25.4
rice, puffed, presweetened, with honey	28	110	1.2	.2	25.7
rice, shredded	28	111	1.5	.1	25.2
rice, with protein concentrates	28	108	11.3	trace	15.5
rice, with wheat gluten	28	109	5.7	.1	21.1
rice flakes	28	110	1.7	.1	24.9
wheat, puffed	28	103	4.2	.4	22.3

Food and measure	gram weight	calories	protein grams	fat grams	carbo-hydrate grams
wheat, puffed, with sugar and honey	28	107	1.7	.6	25.0
wheat, shredded	28	100	2.8	.6	22.6
wheat, shredded, with malt, sugar and salt ..	28	104	2.6	.8	23.2
wheat flakes	28	100	2.9	.4	22.8
wheat germ, toasted	28	111	8.5	3.2	14.0
wheat and malted barley flakes	28	111	2.5	.4	23.9
wheat and malted barley granules	28	111	2.8	.2	23.9
Cervelat, dry, 4 oz.	114	514	28.0	42.9	1.9
Cervelat, soft, 4 oz.	114	350	21.2	27.9	1.8
Chard, Swiss, boiled, drained, 1 cup	191	34	3.4	.4	6.3
Chard, Swiss, raw, trimmed, 1 lb.	454	104	10.0	1.3	19.2
Cheese:					
American, processed, 1 oz.	28	105	6.6	8.5	.5
American, processed, diced, 1 cup	131	484	30.4	39.3	2.5
American, processed, shredded, 1 cup	111	411	25.8	33.3	2.1
American, processed, grated, 1 tablespoon ..	7	23	1.7	2.2	.1
American pimiento, processed, 1 oz.	28	105	6.5	8.6	.5
blue or bleu, 1 oz.	28	104	6.1	8.6	.6
brick, 1 oz.	28	105	6.3	8.6	.5
Camembert, 1 oz.	28	85	5.0	7.0	.5

cheddar, 1 oz.	28	113	7.1	9.1	.6
cheddar, diced, 1 cup	131	521	32.8	42.2	2.8
cheddar, shredded, 1 cup	111	442	27.8	35.7	2.3
cheddar, grated, 1 tablespoon	7	28	1.7	2.2	.1
cottage, creamed, 1 oz.	28	30	3.8	1.2	.8
cottage, creamed, 1 cup	245	260	33.3	10.3	7.1
cottage, uncreamed, 1 oz.	28	24	4.8	.1	.8
cottage, uncreamed, 1 cup	200	172	34.0	.6	5.4
cream, 1 oz.	28	106	2.3	10.7	.6
cream, 1 tablespoon	15	56	1.2	5.6	.3
limburger, 1 oz.	28	98	6.0	7.9	.6
Parmesan, 1 oz.	28	111	10.2	7.4	.8
Parmesan, grated, 1 cup	106	417	38.2	27.6	3.1
Parmesan, grated, 1 tablespoon	7	28	2.5	1.8	.2
Roquefort, 1 oz.	28	104	6.1	8.6	.6
Swiss, natural, 1 cz.	28	105	7.8	7.9	.5
Swiss, processed, 1 oz.	28	101	7.5	7.6	.5
Cheese food, American, processed, 1 oz.	28	92	5.6	6.8	2.0
Cheese spread, American, processed, 1 oz.	28	82	4.5	6.1	2.3
Cheese straws, 1 oz.	28	128	3.2	8.5	9.8
Cherries:					
red sour, fresh, with stems, 1 lb.	454	213	4.4	1.1	52.5
red sour, fresh, pitted, 1 cup	165	96	2.0	.5	23.6

Food and measure	gram weight	calories	protein grams	fat grams	carbo-hydrate grams
red sour, fresh, with pits, 1 cup	160	93	1.9	.5	22.9
red sour, canned in heavy syrup, pitted, 1 cup	235	209	1.9	.5	53.3
red sour, canned, water pack, 1 cup	177	76	1.4	.3	18.9
red sour, frozen, sweetened, 4 oz.	114	128	1.1	.5	15.3
red sour, frozen, unsweetened, 4 oz.	114	63	1.1	.5	6.5
sweet, fresh, with pits, 1 lb.	454	286	5.3	1.2	71.0
sweet, fresh, pitted, 1 cup	165	116	2.1	.5	28.7
sweet, fresh, with pits, 1 cup	160	112	2.1	.5	27.8
sweet, canned in heavy syrup, pitted, 1 cup ..	235	190	2.1	.5	48.2
Cherries, candied, 1 oz.	28	96	.1	.1	24.6
Cherries, candied, 1 average	5	17	trace	trace	4.3
Cherries, maraschino, bottled, 1 oz.	28	33	.1	.1	8.3
Cherries, maraschino, bottled, 1 average ...	7	8	trace	trace	2.1
Chervil, raw, 4 oz.	114	65	3.9	1.0	13.0
Chestnut flour, 4 oz.	114	410	6.9	4.2	86.4
Chestnuts, fresh, in shell, 1 lb.	454	713	10.7	5.5	154.7
Chestnuts, fresh, shelled, 4 oz.	114	220	3.3	1.7	47.8
Chestnuts, dried, shelled, 4 oz.	114	428	7.6	4.7	89.1
Chewing gum, sweetened, 1 oz.	28	90	n.a.	n.a.	27.0
Chewing gum, sweetened, 1 stick	3	9	n.a.	n.a.	2.8

Chicken, canned, boned, 4 oz.	114	226	24.7	13.3	0

Chicken, canned, boned, 4 oz.	114	226	24.7	13.3	0
Chicken, fresh:					
broiled, meat only, 4 oz.	114	155	27.1	4.3	0
cooked, meat only, chopped, 1 cup	143	243	42.9	6.9	0
cooked, meat only, diced, 1 cup	134	228	40.2	6.4	0
fried, ½ breast with bone, 3.3 oz.	94	154	24.8	5.0	1.0
fried, drumstick with bone, 2.1 oz.	59	89	11.8	4.0	trace
roasted, dark meat, 4 oz.	114	210	33.4	7.4	0
roasted, white meat, 4 oz.	114	207	36.8	5.6	0
roasted, meat and skin, 4 oz.	114	283	30.9	16.8	0
stewed, meat only, 4 oz.	114	237	34.2	10.1	0
Chicken, potted, 4 oz.	114	283	9.9	21.9	0
Chicken gizzards, boiled, drained, 4 oz.	114	168	30.8	3.8	.8
Chicken liver, see Liver					
Chicken pot pie, frozen, 8 oz. pie	227	497	15.2	26.1	50.4
Chickpeas, dry, 4 oz.	114	408	23.2	5.4	69.2
Chickpeas, dry, 1 cup	200	720	41.0	9.6	122.0
Chicory, Witloof, see Endive					
Chicory greens, untrimmed, 1 lb.	454	74	6.7	1.1	14.1
Chicory greens, cuts, 1 cup	53	11	.9	.2	2.0
Chicory greens, 10 inner leaves	25	5	.5	trace	1.0
Chili con carne, canned, with beans, 8 oz.	227	302	17.0	13.8	27.7
Chili con carne, canned, without beans, 8 oz.	227	454	23.4	33.6	13.2

Food and measure	gram weight	calories	protein grams	fat grams	carbo-hydrate grams
Chili powder, seasoned, 1 oz.	28	96	4.1	3.5	16.0
Chili powder, seasoned, 1 tablespoon	14	52	2.1	1.8	8.1
Chili sauce, tomato, bottled, 1 cup	247	257	6.2	.7	61.2
Chili sauce, tomato, bottled, 1 tablespoon	16	17	.4	trace	4.0
Chives, raw, 4 oz.	114	32	2.0	.3	6.6
Chocolate, baking-type:					
bitter, unsweetened, 1 oz.	28	143	3.0	15.0	8.2
semi-sweet, 1 oz.	28	144	1.2	10.1	16.2
semi-sweet, chips or morsels, 1 cup	170	862	7.1	60.7	96.9
sweet, 1 oz.	28	150	1.2	9.9	16.4
Chocolate candy, see *Candies*					
Chocolate drinks, see *Cocoa and Milk*					
Chocolate syrup, fudge type, 1 tablespoon	20	66	1.0	2.7	10.8
Chocolate syrup, thin type, 1 tablespoon	20	49	.5	.4	12.5
Chop suey, with meat, canned, 8 oz.	227	141	10.0	7.3	9.5
Chow mein, chicken, canned, 8 oz.	227	86	5.9	.2	16.1
Cider, see *Apple juice*					
Citron, candied, 1 oz.	28	89	trace	.1	22.4
Clam juice or liquor, canned, ½ cup	115	22	2.6	.1	2.4
Clams:					

hard or round, raw, meat only, 8 oz.	227	182	25.2	2.0	13.4
soft, raw, meat only, 8 oz.	227	186	31.8	4.3	3.0
canned, solids and liquid, 4 oz.	114	59	9.0	.8	3.2
canned, drained, 4 oz.	114	112	18.0	2.8	2.2
Cocoa, dry:					
high fat or breakfast, processed, 1 oz.	28	84	4.8	6.7	12.9
high fat or breakfast, processed, 1 tablespoon	6	18	1.0	1.4	2.7
medium fat, processed, 1 oz.	28	74	4.9	5.4	13.7
medium fat, processed, 1 tablespoon	6	16	1.0	1.1	2.9
low medium fat, processed, 1 oz.	28	61	5.4	3.6	14.2
low medium fat, processed, 1 tablespoon	6	13	1.2	.8	3.0
low fat, 1 oz.	28	53	5.7	2.2	16.4
low fat, 1 tablespoon	6	11	1.2	.5	3.5
mix, with nonfat dry milk, 1 oz.	28	102	5.3	.8	20.1
mix, with nonfat dry milk, 1 tablespoon	9	32	1.7	.2	6.4
mix, without milk, 1 oz.	28	98	1.1	.6	25.3
mix, without milk, 1 tablespoon	9	31	.4	.2	8.0
mix, for hot chocolate, 1 oz.	28	111	2.7	3.0	21.0
mix, for hot chocolate, 1 tablespoon	9	35	.8	1.0	6.7
Coconut:					
fresh, meat only, 4 oz.	114	392	4.0	40.0	10.7
fresh, grated, 1 cup	80	277	2.8	28.2	7.5
fresh, shredded, 1 cup	98	339	3.4	34.6	9.2

Food and measure	gram weight	calories	protein grams	fat grams	carbo-hydrate grams
fresh, 1 piece 2 × 2 × ½"	45	156	1.6	15.9	4.2
dried, sweetened, shredded, 4 oz.	114	621	4.1	44.3	60.3
dried, sweetened, shredded, 1 cup	94	515	3.4	36.8	50.0
dried, unsweetened, shredded, 4 oz.	114	751	8.2	73.6	26.1
dried, unsweetened, shredded, 1 cup	94	622	6.8	61.0	21.6
Coconut water (liquid from coconut), 1 cup ..	244	54	.7	.5	11.5
Cod:					
fresh, raw, 4 oz.	114	88	19.9	.3	0
fresh, broiled with butter, 4 oz.	114	194	32.5	6.0	0
canned, 4 oz.	114	97	21.9	.3	0
dehydrated, lightly salted, 4 oz.	114	428	93.3	3.2	0
dried, salted, 4 oz.	114	148	33.1	.8	0
frozen, cakes, reheated, 4 oz.	114	308	10.5	20.4	19.6
frozen, fillets, 4 oz. or 2 average fillets	114	84	18.8	.4	0
frozen, stick, 4 oz. or 5 average sticks	114	276	15.1	10.7	29.1
Coffee, instant, dry, 1 teaspoon	2	3	trace	trace	.7
Coffee, instant, prepared, plain, 1 cup	150	3	trace	trace	.7
Coleslaw, commercial, with French dressing, 4 oz.	114	108	1.4	8.3	8.7
Collards:					

	g	cal			
raw, with stems, 1 lb.	454	181	16.3	3.2	32.7
raw, leaves only, 1 lb.	454	139	14.8	2.5	23.1
boiled, drained, with stems, 1 cup	190	55	5.1	1.1	9.3
boiled, drained, leaves only, 1 cup	190	63	6.8	1.3	9.7
frozen, chopped, boiled, drained, 1 cup	170	51	4.9	.7	9.5
Cookie crumbs, gingersnaps, 1 cup	115	483	6.3	10.2	91.8
Cookie crumbs, graham cracker, 1 cup	86	330	6.9	8.1	63.1
Cookie dough, refrigerated, baked, 1 oz.	28	141	1.1	7.1	18.4
Cookies, baked from mix, 1 oz.:					
brownies, made with nuts, water	28	114	1.4	5.3	16.9
brownies, made with nuts, egg, water	28	121	1.4	5.7	17.9
plain, made with egg, water	28	140	1.4	6.9	18.4
plain, made with milk	28	139	1.0	6.7	18.9
Cookies, packaged commercial, 1 oz.:					
animal crackers	28	122	1.9	2.7	22.7
assorted	28	136	1.4	5.7	20.1
brownies, with nuts, iced, frozen	28	119	1.4	5.8	17.2
butter, thin, rich	28	130	1.7	4.8	20.1
chocolate	28	126	2.0	4.5	20.3
chocolate chip	28	134	1.5	5.9	19.8
coconut bar	28	140	1.8	6.9	18.1
creme sandwich	28	140	1.4	6.4	19.6
fig bar	28	101	1.1	1.6	21.4

Food and measure	gram weight	calories	protein grams	fat grams	carbo-hydrate grams
gingersnaps	28	119	1.6	2.5	22.6
graham crackers	28	109	2.3	2.7	20.8
graham crackers, chocolate coated	28	135	1.4	6.7	19.2
graham crackers, sugar-honey coated	28	116	1.9	3.2	21.6
ladyfingers	28	102	2.2	2.2	18.3
macaroon	28	135	1.5	6.6	18.7
marshmallow	28	116	1.1	3.7	20.5
molasses	28	120	1.8	3.0	21.5
oatmeal, with raisins	28	123	1.8	4.4	20.8
peanut	28	134	2.8	5.4	19.0
raisin	28	107	1.2	1.5	22.9
shortbread	28	141	2.0	6.5	18.4
sugar wafers	28	137	1.4	5.5	20.8
vanilla wafers	28	131	1.5	4.6	21.1
Corn, sweet:					
fresh, on cob, without husks, 1 lb.	454	240	8.7	2.5	55.1
fresh, on cob, boiled, drained, 1 ear 5"	140	71	2.6	.8	16.4
fresh, kernels, boiled, drained, 1 cup	166	138	5.2	1.6	31.2
canned, kernels, boiled, drained, 1 cup	173	145	4.5	1.4	34.3
canned, kernels, vacuum-packed, heated, 1 cup	212	176	5.3	1.1	43.5

canned, cream-style, heated, 1 cup	253	207	5.3	1.5	50.6
frozen, on cob, 1 ear (3½ oz.)	100	82	3.1	.5	19.1
frozen, kernels, boiled, drained, 1 cup	182	144	5.5	.9	34.2
Corn bread mix, made with egg, milk, 2 oz.	57	132	3.6	4.8	18.7
Corn flour, 4 oz.	114	417	8.8	2.9	87.1
Corn grits, degermed, dry, ¼ cup	40	145	3.5	.3	31.2
Corn grits, degermed, cooked, 1 cup	242	123	2.9	2.4	26.6
Cornmeal, cooked, 1 cup	240	120	2.6	.5	25.7
Cornmeal, white or yellow, dry form, 4 oz.:					
whole ground, unbolted	114	403	10.4	4.4	83.6
bolted	114	411	10.2	3.9	84.5
degermed	114	413	8.9	1.4	88.9
self-rising, whole ground	114	393	9.7	3.4	81.5
self-rising, degermed	114	395	8.6	1.2	85.3
Corn muffin, baked from mix, 2 oz.:					
made with egg, milk	57	185	3.9	6.0	28.5
made with egg, water	57	169	2.6	4.4	29.6
Cornstarch, 1 cup	130	470	.4	trace	113.9
Cornstarch, 1 tablespoon	8	28	trace	trace	7.0
Cowpeas, immature seeds:					
raw, in pods, 1 lb.	454	317	22.5	2.0	54.4
raw, shelled, 1 lb.	454	576	40.8	3.6	98.9
fresh, boiled, drained, 1 cup	160	173	13.0	1.3	29.0

Food and measure	gram weight	calories	protein grams	fat grams	carbo-hydrate grams
canned, with liquid, 4 oz.	114	80	5.7	.3	14.1
frozen, boiled, drained, 1 cup	142	185	12.6	.6	33.5
Cowpeas, mature seeds, dry, 1 cup	170	583	38.8	2.6	104.9
Cowpeas, mature seeds, cooked, 1 cup	248	188	12.6	7.4	34.2
Crab:					
fresh, steamed in shell, 1 lb.	454	202	37.7	4.1	1.1
fresh, steamed, meat only, 4 oz.	114	105	19.6	2.2	.6
canned, meat only, 4 oz.	114	115	19.7	2.8	1.2
canned, meat only, 1 cup	170	172	29.6	4.2	1.9
Crabapples, raw, whole, 1 lb.	454	284	1.7	1.3	74.3
Crabapples, raw, flesh only, 4 oz.	114	77	.5	.3	20.2
Cracker crumbs, see *Cookie crumbs*					
Cracker meal, 4 oz.	114	497	10.4	14.8	80.1
Cracker meal, 1 tablespoon	10	44	.9	1.3	7.1
Crackers, commercial packaged, 1 oz.:					
barbecue flavor	28	142	1.9	7.5	18.0
butter	28	130	2.0	5.0	19.1
cheese	28	136	3.2	6.0	17.1
oyster	28	112	2.8	2.8	19.8
peanut butter-cheese sandwich	28	139	4.3	6.8	15.9

saltines	28	123	2.6	3.4	20.3
soda	28	124	2.6	3.7	20.0
whole wheat	28	114	2.4	3.9	19.3
zwieback	28	121	2.8	2.8	21.8
Cranberries:					
fresh, whole, 1 lb.	454	200	1.7	3.0	47.0
fresh, without stems, 1 cup	115	53	.5	.8	12.4
dehydrated, 1 oz.	28	104	.8	1.9	23.9
Cranberry juice cocktail, bottled, 6 oz. glass	188	122	trace	.2	31.0
Cranberry-orange relish, uncooked, 1 cup	280	498	1.1	1.1	127.1
Cranberry sauce, canned, sweet, strained, 1 oz.	28	41	trace	trace	10.7
Cranberry sauce, canned, sweet, strained, 1 cup	271	396	.3	.5	101.6
Crayfish, raw, in shell, 1 lb.	454	39	7.9	.3	.7
Crayfish, raw, meat only, 1 lb.	454	327	66.2	2.3	5.4
Cream, dairy:					
half and half, 1 cup	242	324	7.7	28.3	11.1
half and half, 1 tablespoon	15	20	.5	1.8	.7
light, table or coffee, 1 cup	240	506	7.2	59.4	10.4
light, table or coffee, 1 tablespoon	15	32	.4	3.1	.6
whipping, light, 1 cup unwhipped	239	717	6.0	74.8	8.6
whipping, light, 1 tablespoon unwhipped	15	45	.4	4.7	.5
whipping, light, 1 cup whipped	119	357	3.0	37.2	4.3
whipping, light, 1 tablespoon whipped	7	23	.2	2.4	.3

Food and measure	gram weight	calories	protein grams	fat grams	carbo-hydrate grams
whipping, heavy, 1 cup unwhipped	238	837	5.2	89.4	7.4
whipping, heavy, 1 tablespoon unwhipped ..	15	53	.3	5.6	.5
whipping, heavy, 1 cup whipped	119	419	2.6	44.7	3.7
whipping, heavy, 1 tablespoon whipped	7	27	.2	2.8	.3
Cream, sour, 1 cup	230	485	7.0	47.0	10.0
Cream, sour, 1 tablespoon	12	26	.3	2.0	1.0
Cream products, imitation:					
creamer, powdered, 1 tablespoon	6	30	.6	1.5	3.6
creamer, frozen, liquid, 1 tablespoon	15	20	trace	2.0	2.0
sour cream dressing, 1 tablespoon	12	20	trace	2.0	1.0
Cress, garden:					
raw, untrimmed, 1 lb.	454	103	8.4	2.3	17.7
boiled in little water, drained, 1 cup	200	46	3.8	1.2	7.6
boiled in large amount water, drained, 1 cup	200	44	3.6	1.2	7.2
Cress, water, see *Watercress*					
Croaker, Atlantic, baked, 4 oz.	114	152	27.7	3.6	0
Croaker, Atlantic, whole, 1 lb.	454	148	27.4	3.4	0
Cucumber:					
fresh, with skin, 1 lb.	454	65	3.9	.4	14.7
fresh, with skin, 1 medium, 7½ × 2"	207	31	1.2	.2	6.9

fresh, pared, 1 medium, 7½ × 2"	207	29	1.2	.2	6.6
fresh, sliced, pared, 6 slices, ⅛ × 2"	50	7	.3	trace	1.6
fresh, diced, pared, 1 cup	144	20	.9	.1	4.6
pickled, see *Pickles*					
Currants:					
black, fresh, with stems, 1 lb.	454	240	7.6	.4	58.2
black, fresh, without stems, 1 cup	114	60	1.9	.1	14.5
red or white, fresh, with stems, 1 lb.	454	220	6.2	.9	53.2
red or white, fresh, without stems, 1 cup	114	55	1.5	.2	13.3
Custard, see *Pudding* and *Pies*					
Dandelion greens, raw, fully trimmed, 1 lb.	454	204	12.2	3.2	41.7
Dandelion greens, boiled, drained, 1 cup	180	59	3.6	1.1	11.5
Date, Chinese, see *Jujube*					
Dates, domestic, natural and dry:					
with pits, 1 lb.	454	1081	8.7	2.0	287.7
pitted, 1 lb.	454	1243	10.0	2.3	330.7
pitted, 4 average (about 1 oz.)	26	71	.8	.1	18.9
pitted, chopped, 1 cup	174	477	3.8	.9	126.8
pitted, chopped, 1 cup loosely packed	142	389	3.1	.7	103.5
Dewberries, see *Blackberries*					
Dock or sorrel, raw, with stems, 1 lb.	454	89	6.7	1.0	17.8
Dock or sorrel, boiled, drained, 1 cup	200	38	3.2	.4	7.8

Food and measure	gram weight	calories	protein grams	fat grams	carbohydrate grams
Doughnuts, cake type, 1 average	32	125	1.5	5.9	16.4
Doughnuts, cake type, 1 oz.	28	111	1.3	5.3	14.6
Doughnuts, yeast-leavened, 1 oz.	28	117	1.8	7.7	10.7
Duck, domestic, roasted, meat only, 4 oz.	114	352	25.8	26.7	0
Duck, wild, raw, meat only, 4 oz.	114	157	24.3	5.9	0
Eel, American, meat only, raw, 4 oz.	114	264	18.0	20.7	0
Eel, smoked, 4 oz.	114	376	21.2	31.7	0
Egg, chicken:					
raw, whole, 1 large	50	81	6.4	5.7	.4
raw, white from 1 large egg	33	17	3.6	trace	.3
raw, yolk from 1 large egg	17	59	2.7	5.2	.4
boiled, 1 large	50	81	6.4	5.7	.4
cooked with ½ tablespoon butter, 1 large ..	50	108	6.9	8.6	.2
poached, 1 large	50	81	6.3	5.8	.4
dried, whole, 2 tablespoons	14	83	6.6	5.8	.5
dried, whole, ½ cup	54	320	25.4	22.2	2.2
dried, white, powdered, 2 tablespoons	14	52	11.2	trace	.8
dried, yolk, 2 tablespoons	14	93	4.6	7.9	.4
Egg, duck, raw, whole, 1 average	75	143	10.0	10.9	.5

	Grams	Calories	Protein	Fat	Carbohydrate
Eggnog, dairy-packaged, 6% butterfat, 1 cup ..	250	160	4.1	8.3	17.3
Eggnog, dairy-packaged, 8% butterfat, 1 cup ..	255	186	4.2	11.0	17.6
Eggplant, boiled, drained, 1 cup	200	38	2.0	.4	8.2
Eggplant, raw, whole, 1 lb.	454	92	4.4	.7	20.6
Eggplant, raw, diced, 1 cup	398	50	2.4	.4	11.2
Elderberries, raw, with stems, 1 lb.	454	307	11.1	2.1	69.9
Elderberries, raw, without stems, 4 oz.	114	82	2.9	.6	18.6
Endive, French or Belgian:					
fresh, whole, 1 lb.	454	80	6.8	.4	16.4
fresh, 10 small leaves	25	5	.4	trace	1.0
fresh, cut, 1 cup	50	10	.8	trace	2.0
Escarole:					
fresh, untrimmed, 1 lb.	454	80	6.8	.4	16.4
fresh, 4 large outer leaves	100	20	1.7	.1	4.1
fresh, 7 small leaves	20	4	.3	trace	.8
fresh, shredded, 1 cup	71	14	1.2	.1	2.9
Farina, see Cereal, cooking-type					
Fennel leaves, raw, untrimmed, 1 lb.	454	118	11.8	1.7	21.5
Fennel leaves, raw, trimmed, 4 oz.	114	32	3.2	.5	5.8
Figs:					
raw, 1 lb.	454	363	5.4	1.4	92.1
canned in heavy syrup, whole, 1 cup ...	252	213	1.3	.5	55.2

Food and measure	gram weight	calories	protein grams	fat grams	carbo- hydrate grams
canned, 3 figs, 2 tablespoons heavy syrup ..	115	96	.6	.2	25.0
dried, uncooked, 4 oz.	114	311	4.9	1.5	78.4
dried, uncooked, 1 large (2" × 1")	21	57	.9	.3	14.5
candied, 1 oz.	28	85	.9	trace	20.9
Filberts, in shell, 1 lb.	454	1323	26.3	130.2	34.9
Filberts, shelled, 4 oz.	114	719	14.3	70.7	18.9
Filberts, 10–12 nuts	15	95	1.9	9.4	2.5
Finnan haddie, flesh only, raw, 1 lb.	454	467	105.2	1.8	0
Fish, see individual listings					
Fish bites, breaded, frozen, cooked, 4 oz.	114	268	11.2	13.8	24.6
Fish cakes, breaded, frozen, cooked, 4 oz.	114	308	10.5	20.4	19.6
Fish flakes, canned, 1 oz.	28	31	7.0	.2	0
Fish flour (from whole fish), 1 oz.	28	95	22.1	.1	0
Fish flour (from fish fillets), 1 oz.	28	113	26.4	trace	0
Fish sticks, breaded, frozen, cooked, 4 oz.	114	201	18.9	10.1	7.1
Flounder, fillets, raw, 4 oz.	114	89	18.9	.9	0
Flounder, raw, whole, 1 lb.	454	118	25.0	1.2	0
Flour (see also individual listings):					
buckwheat, whole grain, sifted, 1 cup	100	335	11.7	2.4	72.9
buckwheat, dark, sifted, 1 cup	100	333	11.7	2.5	72.0

buckwheat, light, sifted, 1 cup	100	347	6.4	1.2	79.5
carob or Saint-John's-bread, 3½ oz.	100	180	4.5	1.4	80.7
rye, dark, stirred, 1 cup	127	415	20.7	3.3	86.5
rye, light, unsifted, 1 cup	100	357	9.4	1.0	77.9
soybean, defatted, stirred, 1 cup	120	391	56.4	1.8	45.7
soybean, defatted, sifted, 1 cup	100	326	47.0	.9	38.1
soybean, high fat, 3½ oz.	100	380	41.2	12.1	33.3
wheat, all purpose, unsifted, 1 cup	126	458	13.2	1.3	95.9
wheat, all purpose, sifted, 1 cup	115	419	12.1	1.2	87.5
wheat, bread, unsifted, 1 cup	123	449	14.5	1.4	91.9
wheat, bread, sifted, 1 cup	117	427	13.8	1.3	87.4
wheat, cake, unsifted, 1 cup	111	404	8.3	.9	88.1
wheat, cake, sifted, 1 cup	100	364	7.5	.8	79.4
wheat, gluten, unsifted, 1 cup	135	510	55.9	2.6	63.7
wheat, gluten, sifted, 1 cup	131	491	53.8	2.5	61.4
wheat, self-rising, unsifted, 1 cup	127	447	11.8	1.2	94.2
wheat, self-rising, sifted, 1 cup	106	373	9.8	1.1	78.7
wheat, whole, stirred, 1 cup	137	456	18.2	2.7	97.3
Frankfurters:					
raw, average, all samples, 4 oz.	114	350	14.2	31.3	2.0
raw, all meat, 4 oz.	114	336	14.9	28.9	2.8
raw, with cereal added, 4 oz.	114	281	16.3	23.4	.2
raw, with nonfat dry milk added, 4 oz.	114	340	14.9	29.0	3.9

Food and measure	gram weight	calories	protein grams	fat grams	carbo-hydrate grams
cooked, all meat, 1 average (8 per lb.)	56	170	6.9	15.2	.9
canned, 4 oz. ..	114	251	15.2	20.5	.2
Frog's legs, raw, whole, 1 lb. ..	454	215	48.3	.9	0
Frog's legs, raw, meat only, 4 oz.	114	83	18.6	.3	0
Frosting, see *Icing*					
Fruit, see individual listings					
Fruit, mixed, frozen, sweetened, 8 oz.	227	250	1.0	.2	63.8
Fruit cocktail, canned:					
with heavy syrup, 8 oz.	227	173	.9	.3	44.7
with heavy syrup, 1 cup	256	195	1.0	.3	50.4
water pack, 8 oz.	227	84	.9	.3	22.0
Fruit for salad, canned:					
with heavy syrup, 8 oz.	227	170	.7	.3	44.0
with heavy syrup, 1 cup	246	185	.7	.2	47.7
water pack, 8 oz.	227	80	.9	.3	20.7
Fruit salad, dairy packaged, 8 oz.	227	136	1.4	.4	29.8
Garbanzos, see *Chickpeas*					
Garlic, cloves, whole, 2 oz.	57	68	3.1	.1	15.4
Garlic, cloves, peeled, 5 cloves	10	14	.6	trace	3.1

Food	Weight (g)	Calories	Protein	Fat	Carbohydrate
Gelatin:					
unflavored, dry, 1 package	7	25	6.0	trace	0
unflavored, dry, 1 tablespoon	10	33	8.5	trace	0
flavored dessert mix, dry, 3 oz. package	85	315	8.0	0	74.8
flavored dessert mix, made with water, 1 cup	240	142	4.0	0	33.8
Ginger, candied, crystallized, 1 oz.	28	97	trace	trace	24.6
Ginger root, fresh, 1 oz.	28	14	.4	.3	2.7
Goose, roasted, meat and skin, 4 oz.	114	503	26.1	43.4	0
Goose, roasted, meat only, 4 oz.	114	266	38.6	11.2	0
Gooseberries:					
fresh, 1 lb.	454	177	3.6	.9	44.0
fresh, 1 cup	150	59	1.2	.3	14.6
canned with heavy syrup, 8 oz.	227	204	1.1	.2	52.2
canned, water pack, 8 oz.	227	59	1.1	.2	15.0
Grapefruit, canned, in syrup, 1 cup	256	179	1.5	.3	45.6
Grapefruit, canned, water pack, 1 cup	246	74	1.5	.2	18.7
Grapefruit, fresh:					
pink or red, seeded, whole, 1 lb.	454	87	1.1	.2	22.6
pink or red, seedless, whole, 1 lb.	454	93	1.2	.2	24.1
pink or red, ½ medium (4½" diameter)	285	58	.7	.1	15.1
pink or red, sections, 1 cup	200	80	1.0	.2	20.8
white, seeded, whole, 1 lb.	454	84	1.0	.2	22.0
white, seedless, whole, 1 lb.	454	87	1.1	.2	22.4

Food and measure	gram weight	calories	protein grams	fat grams	carbo- hydrate grams
white, seeded, ½ medium (4½" diameter) ..	285	52	.6	.1	13.8
white, seedless, ½ medium (4½" diameter) ..	285	53	.7	.1	12.6
white, sections, 1 cup	200	80	1.0	.2	20.9
Grapefruit juice:					
fresh, 6 oz. glass	185	72	.9	.1	16.9
canned, sweetened, 6 oz. glass	188	100	.9	.1	24.0
canned, unsweetened, 6 oz. glass	185	76	.9	.1	18.1
frozen, sweetened, diluted, 6 oz. glass ...	175	82	.7	.2	19.9
frozen, unsweetened, diluted, 6 oz. glass ...	175	72	.9	.2	17.2
dehydrated, crystals, 1 tablespoon	8	30	.4	.1	7.2
dehydrated, diluted, 6 oz. glass	185	74	.9	.2	17.7
Grapefruit-orange juice, see *Orange-grapefruit juice*					
Grapefruit peel, candied, 1 oz.	28	90	.1	.1	22.9
Grape juice:					
canned, 6 oz. glass	185	122	.4	trace	30.7
frozen, sweetened, diluted, 6 oz. glass ...	185	98	.4	trace	24.6
Grape juice drink, canned, 6 oz. glass	185	99	.3	trace	25.3
Grapes, American type (Concord, Delaware, etc.):					

Food	Grams	Calories	Protein	Fat	Carbohydrate
fresh, 1 lb.	454	197	3.7	2.9	44.9
fresh, whole, 1 cup	153	66	1.2	1.0	15.0
Grapes, European type (Malaga, Thompson seedless, etc.):					
fresh, 1 lb.	454	270	2.4	1.2	69.8
fresh, whole, 1 cup	160	95	.9	.4	24.6
Grapes, seedless, canned, water pack, 1 cup ..	200	102	1.0	.2	27.2
Grapes, seedless, canned in heavy syrup, 1 cup	200	154	1.0	.2	40.0
Grouper, raw, meat only, 4 oz.	114	99	21.9	.6	0
Grouper, raw, whole, 1 lb.	454	170	37.6	1.0	0
Guava, fresh:					
common, whole, with stems, 1 lb.	454	273	3.5	2.6	66.0
common, trimmed, 4 oz.	114	70	.9	.7	17.0
common, 1 small	80	48	.6	.5	11.7
strawberry, with stems, 1 lb.	454	289	4.4	2.7	70.2
strawberry, trimmed, 4 oz.	114	74	1.1	.7	17.9
Guinea hen, raw, whole, ready-to-cook, 1 lb. ...	454	594	88.0	24.4	0
Gum, see *Chewing gum*					
Haddock:					
raw, whole, 1 lb.	454	172	39.8	.2	0
raw, meat only, 4 oz.	114	90	20.8	.1	0
fresh, fillet, breaded, fried, 3½ oz.	100	165	19.6	6.4	5.8

Food and measure	gram weight	calories	protein grams	fat grams	carbohydrate grams
frozen, fillet, 4 oz.	114	88	20.8	.1	0
smoked, 4 oz.	114	117	26.3	.5	0
Halibut, Atlantic or Pacific:					
raw, whole, 1 lb.	454	268	55.9	3.2	0
fresh, broiled with butter, 4 oz.	114	195	28.7	8.0	0
frozen, steak, 4 oz.	114	144	21.2	6.0	0
smoked, 4 oz.	114	254	23.6	17.0	0
Ham, deviled, canned, 2 oz.	57	200	7.8	18.4	0
Ham, meat only:					
boiled, 4 oz.	114	266	21.6	19.4	0
fresh, medium-fat, roasted, 4 oz.	114	426	26.2	34.8	0
light-cured, medium fat, roasted, 4 oz.	114	329	23.8	25.2	0
light-cured, lean, roasted, 4 oz.	114	213	28.8	10.0	0
long-cured, country style, medium fat, 4 oz. ..	114	443	19.3	39.9	0
long-cured, country style, lean, 4 oz. ...	114	353	22.2	28.5	0
picnic, medium fat, roasted, 4 oz.	114	368	25.5	28.7	0
picnic, lean, roasted, 4 oz.	114	241	32.4	11.3	0
Ham, spiced, canned, 2 oz.	57	168	8.5	14.2	.7
Hamburger, see Beef, ground					
Hazelnuts, see Filberts					

	Grams	Calories	Protein	Fat	Carbohydrate
Headcheese, 4 oz.	114	305	17.7	25.1	1.1
Heart, fresh, 4 oz.:					
beef, lean, braised	114	214	35.7	6.5	.8
calf, braised	114	237	31.7	10.4	2.0
chicken, simmered	114	197	28.8	8.2	.1
lamb, braised	114	296	33.6	16.4	1.1
turkey, simmered	114	246	25.8	15.0	.3
Herring:					
Atlantic, raw, whole, 1 lb.	454	407	40.0	26.1	0
Atlantic, raw, meat only, 4 oz.	114	200	19.6	12.8	0
Pacific, raw, meat only, 4 oz.	114	111	19.8	2.9	0
canned, plain, with liquid, 4 oz.	114	236	22.6	15.4	0
canned, with tomato sauce, 4 oz.	114	200	17.9	11.9	4.2
pickled, Bismark type, 4 oz.	114	253	23.1	17.1	0
salted or brined, 4 oz.	114	247	21.5	17.2	0
smoked, bloaters, 4 oz.	114	222	22.6	14.1	0
smoked, hard, 4 oz.	114	340	41.8	17.9	0
smoked, kippered, 4 oz.	114	239	25.2	14.6	0
Hickory nuts, in shell, 1 lb.	454	1068	21.0	109.1	20.3
Hickory nuts, shelled, 4 oz.	114	763	15.0	78.0	14.5
Hominy, see *Corn grits*					
Honey, strained or extracted, 1 cup	326	991	1.0	0	268.3
Honey, strained or extracted, 1 tablespoon	21	64	trace	0	17.3

Food and measure	gram weight	calories	protein grams	fat grams	carbohydrate grams
Honeydew melon, fresh:					
whole, 1 lb.	454	94	2.3	.9	22.0
1 wedge, 2 × 7″	150	49	1.2	.5	11.5
diced, 1 cup	168	55	1.3	.5	12.9
Horseradish, prepared, 1 oz.	28	11	.4	.1	2.7
Horseradish, raw, whole, 1 lb.	454	288	10.6	1.0	65.2
Horseradish, raw, pared, 1 oz.	28	25	.9	.1	5.6
Ice cream and frozen custard:					
regular, about 10% fat, 1 cup	133	257	6.0	14.1	27.7
regular, about 12% fat, 1 cup	133	275	5.3	16.6	27.4
rich, about 16% fat, 1 cup	148	329	3.8	23.8	26.6
Ice cream cone, 1 oz.	28	107	2.8	.7	22.1
Ice cream cone, 1 average	5	19	.5	.1	3.9
Ice milk, hardened, 1 cup	131	199	6.3	6.7	29.3
Ice milk, soft-serve, 1 cup	175	266	8.4	8.9	39.2
Ices, water, lime, 1 cup	180	140	.7	trace	58.7
Icing, cake, mix, made with water, table fat:					
chocolate fudge, 1 oz.	28	107	.6	4.1	19.0
creamy fudge, 1 oz.	28	109	.7	4.3	18.7

	grams	calories	protein	fat	carbohydrate
Jackfruit, raw, flesh only, 4 oz.	114	111	1.5	.3	28.8
Jackfruit, raw, whole, 1 lb.	454	124	1.7	.4	32.3
Jack mackeral, raw, meat only, 4 oz.	114	162	24.5	6.4	0
Jams and preserves, all flavors, 1 oz.	28	77	.2	trace	19.8
Jams and preserves, all flavors, 1 tablespoon	20	54	.1	trace	14.0
Jellies, all flavors, 1 oz.	28	77	trace	trace	20.0
Jellies, all flavors, 1 tablespoon	20	55	trace	trace	14.3
Jerusalem artichoke, raw, pared, 4 oz.	114	76	2.6	.1	18.9
Juices, see individual listings					
Jujube (Chinese date):					
fresh, whole, 1 lb.	454	443	5.1	.8	116.4
fresh, seeded, 4 oz.	114	119	1.4	.2	31.3
dried, whole, 1 lb.	454	1159	14.9	4.4	297.1
dried, seeded, 4 oz.	114	325	4.2	1.2	83.5
Kale:					
raw, with stems, 1 lb.	454	128	14.1	2.7	20.1
raw, leaves only, 4 oz.	114	60	6.8	.9	10.2
boiled, drained, leaves and stems, 1 cup	110	31	3.5	.8	4.4
frozen, boiled, drained, 1 cup	184	57	5.5	.9	9.9
Kidney:					
beef, raw, 4 oz.	114	147	17.5	7.6	1.0

Food and measure	gram weight	calories	protein grams	fat grams	carbo-hydrate grams
beef, braised, 4 oz.	114	286	37.4	13.6	.9
calf, raw, 4 oz.	114	128	18.8	5.2	.1
hog, raw, 4 oz.	114	120	18.5	4.1	1.2
lamb, raw, 4 oz.	114	119	19.1	3.7	1.0
Kingfish, raw, meat only, 4 oz. ..	114	119	20.8	3.4	0
Kingfish, raw, whole, 1 lb.	454	210	36.5	6.0	0
Kippers, see *Herring*					
Knockwurst, 4 oz.	114	317	16.1	26.4	2.5
Kohlrabi:					
raw, whole, without leaves, 1 lb.	454	96	6.6	.3	21.9
raw, pared, 4 oz.	114	33	2.3	.1	7.5
boiled, drained, 1 cup	155	37	2.6	.2	8.2
Kumquats:					
fresh, whole, 1 lb.	454	274	3.8	.4	72.1
fresh, with seeds, 4 oz.	114	74	1.0	.1	19.4
fresh, 4 average	60	39	.5	trace	10.3
Lake herring (cisco), raw, meat only, 4 oz.	114	109	20.1	2.6	0
Lake herring (cisco), raw, whole, 1 lb.	454	226	41.8	5.4	0
Lake trout, raw, meat only, 4 oz.	114	191	20.8	11.3	0

Lake trout, raw, whole, 1 lb.	454	282	30.7	16.8	0
Lake trout (siscowet), raw:					
under 6.5 lbs., whole, 1 lb.	454	404	24.0	33.4	0
under 6.5 lbs., meat only, 4 oz.	114	273	16.2	22.6	0
over 6.5 lbs., whole, 1 lb.	454	856	12.9	88.8	0
over 6.5 lbs., meat only, 4 oz.	114	594	8.9	61.7	0
Lamb, fresh, choice grade:					
chop, loin, 4.8 oz. with bone, broiled, lean and fat	112	402	24.6	32.9	0
chop, loin, 4.8 oz. with bone, broiled, lean only	74	140	20.8	5.5	0
chop, rib, boned, broiled, lean and fat, 4 oz.	114	462	22.8	40.4	0
chop, rib, boned, broiled, lean only, 4 oz.	114	239	30.8	11.9	0
leg, roasted, lean and fat, 4 oz.	114	318	28.8	21.5	0
leg, roasted, lean only, 4 oz.	114	212	32.7	8.0	0
shoulder, roasted, lean and fat, 4 oz.	114	385	24.7	31.0	0
shoulder, roasted, lean only, 4 oz.	114	234	32.6	11.4	0
Lambsquarter, boiled, drained, 1 cup	200	64	6.4	1.4	10.0
Lambsquarter, raw, fully trimmed, 1 lb.	454	195	19.1	3.6	33.1
Lard, 1 cup	205	1849	0	205.0	0
Lard, 1 tablespoon	13	117	0	13.0	0
Leeks:					
raw, untrimmed, 1 lb.	454	123	5.2	.7	26.4
raw, bulb and lower leaf, 4 oz.	114	59	2.5	.3	12.7
raw, 3 average	100	52	2.2	.3	11.2
Lemonade, frozen, sweetened, diluted, 1 cup	242	106	.2	trace	27.6

Food and measure	gram weight	calories	protein grams	fat grams	carbohydrate grams
Lemon juice, unsweetened:					
fresh, ½ cup	123	31	.6	.2	9.8
fresh, 1 tablespoon	15	4	.1	trace	1.2
canned or bottled, ½ cup	122	28	.5	.1	9.3
canned or bottled, 1 tablespoon	15	3	.1	trace	1.1
frozen, single-strength, ½ cup	122	27	.4	.2	8.8
Lemon peel, candied, 1 oz.	28	88	.1	.1	22.6
Lemon peel, fresh, from 1 average lemon	34	n.a.	.5	.1	5.4
Lemons, 1 average (2⅛" diameter)	110	20	.8	.2	5.8
Lemons, fresh, with peel, 1 lb.	454	90	5.4	1.3	48.1
Lentils:					
whole, dry, 4 oz.	114	386	28.0	1.2	68.2
whole, dry, 1 cup	190	646	46.9	2.1	114.2
whole, cooked, drained, 1 cup	202	214	15.8	trace	39.0
split, dry, 4 oz.	114	391	28.0	1.0	70.1
Lettuce, fresh:					
Boston or bibb, untrimmed, 1 lb.	454	47	4.0	.7	8.4
Boston or bibb, 1 head (4" diameter)	220	31	2.6	.4	5.5
iceberg, untrimmed, 1 lb. head (4¾" diam)	454	56	3.9	.4	12.5
iceberg, 3 average leaves	45	6	.4	trace	1.3
iceberg, chopped, 1 cup	59	8	.5	.1	1.7
iceberg, chunks, 1 cup	74	10	.7	.1	2.1

looseleaf, untrimmed, 1 lb.	454	52	3.8	.9	10.2
looseleaf, 2 'large leaves	50	9	.6	.1	1.8
romaine, untrimmed, 1 lb.	454	52	3.8	.9	10.2
romaine, 3 leaves (8" long)	28	5	.4	.1	1.0
Lichee nuts:					
raw, in shell, 1 lb.	454	174	2.4	.8	44.6
dry, in shell, 1 lb.	454	578	7.9	2.5	147.6
dry, shelled, 6 average	15	41	.6	.2	10.6
Lima beans, see Beans, lima					
Limeade, frozen, sweetened, diluted, 1 cup	247	101	trace	trace	27.2
Lime juice, unsweetened:					
fresh, ½ cup	123	32	.4	.1	11.1
fresh, 1 tablespoon	15	4	trace	trace	1.4
canned or bottled, ½ cup	123	32	.4	.1	11.1
canned or bottled, 1 tablespoon	15	4	trace	trace	1.4
Limes, fresh, with peel, 1 lb.	454	107	2.7	.8	36.2
Limes, fresh, 1 average (1½" long)	68	19	.5	.1	6.5
Liquor, see Alcoholic beverages					
Liver, fresh:					
beef, fried, 4 oz.	114	260	29.9	12.0	6.0
calf, fried, 4 oz.	114	296	33.5	15.0	4.5
chicken, simmered, 4 oz.	114	187	30.1	5.0	3.5
lamb, broiled, 4 oz.	114	296	36.6	14.1	3.2
pig, fried, 4 oz.	114	273	33.9	13.0	2.8
turkey, simmered, 4 oz.	114	197	31.6	5.4	3.5
Liver paste, see *Pâté de foie gras*					

Food and measure	gram weight	calories	protein grams	fat grams	carbo-hydrate grams
Liverwurst, fresh, 4 oz.	114	350	18.5	29.2	2.0
Liverwurst, smoked, 4 oz.	114	364	16.9	31.2	2.6
Lobster, northern:					
raw, whole (in shell), 1 lb.	454	107	19.9	2.2	.6
fresh, cooked in shell, 1 lb.	454	112	22.0	1.8	.4
fresh or canned, cooked, meat only, 4 oz. ..	114	108	21.2	1.7	.3
Lobster paste, canned, 1 oz.	28	51	5.9	2.7	.4
Loganberries:					
fresh, untrimmed, 1 lb.	454	267	4.3	2.6	64.2
fresh, trimmed, 1 cup	145	90	1.5	.9	21.6
canned, water pack, 4 oz.	114	45	.8	.5	10.7
canned, with heavy syrup, 4 oz. ..	114	101	.7	.5	25.2
Loquats, flesh only, 4 oz.	114	54	.5	.2	14.1
Loquats, fresh, whole, 1 lb.	454	168	1.4	.7	43.3
Luncheon meat, see individual listings					
Lychee nuts, see *Lichee nuts*					
Macademia nuts:					
in shell, 1 lb.	454	972	11.0	100.7	22.4
shelled, 4 oz.	114	784	8.6	81.2	18.0
shelled, 6 average	15	104	1.2	10.7	2.4
Macaroni, elbow:					
dry, 1 cup	136	502	17.0	1.6	102.3

cooked 8–10 minutes, drained, 1 cup	130	192	6.5	.6	39.1
cooked 14–20 minutes, drained, 1 cup	140	155	4.8	.6	32.2
Macaroni and cheese, canned, 8 oz. can	227	215	8.8	9.1	24.3
Macaroni and cheese, canned, 1 cup	240	228	9.4	9.6	25.7
Mackerel:					
Atlantic, raw, whole, 1 lb.	454	468	46.5	29.9	0
Atlantic, broiled with butter, meat only, 4 oz.	114	268	24.7	17.9	0
Atlantic, canned, with liquid, 4 oz.	114	208	21.9	12.6	0
Pacific, raw, dressed, 1 lb.	454	519	71.5	23.8	0
Pacific, canned with liquid, 4 oz.	114	204	23.9	11.3	0
salted, meat only, 4 oz.	114	345	21.0	28.5	0
smoked, meat only, 4 oz.	114	248	27.0	14.7	0
Malt, dry, 1 oz.	28	104	3.7	.5	21.9
Malt extract, dried, 1 oz.	28	104	1.7	trace	25.3
Mandarin oranges, see *Tangerines*					
Mangoes, fresh:					
whole, 1 lb.	454	201	2.1	1.2	51.1
whole, 1 average (3¾″ long)	303	134	1.4	.8	34.1
diced, 1 cup	163	108	1.1	.7	27.4
Maple syrup, see *Syrups*					
Margarine:					
1 cup or ½ lb.	227	1633	1.4	183.5	.9
1 tablespoon	14	101	.1	11.3	trace
whipped, 1 cup	152	1094	.9	123.1	.6
Marmalade, citrus, 1 tablespoon	20	51	.1	trace	14.0

247

Food and measure	gram weight	calories	protein grams	fat grams	carbo-hydrate grams
Mayonnaise, see *Salad dressings*					
Meat, see individual listings					
Melon, see individual listings					
Melon balls, in syrup, frozen, 8 oz.	227	141	1.4	.2	35.6
Melon balls, in syrup, frozen, 1 cup	231	143	1.4	.2	36.3
Milk, canned, concentrated:					
condensed, sweetened, ½ cup	153	491	12.4	13.3	83.1
evaporated, unsweetened, ½ cup	126	173	8.8	9.9	12.2
Milk, chocolate, canned or dairy-packed:					
made with whole milk, 1 cup	250	213	8.5	8.5	27.5
made with skim milk, 1 cup	250	190	8.2	5.7	27.2
Milk, cow's, fresh:					
whole, 3.5% fat, 1 cup	244	159	8.5	8.5	11.9
whole, 3.7% fat, 1 cup	244	161	8.5	9.0	11.9
buttermilk, cultured, 1 cup	244	88	8.8	2.4	12.4
half and half, see *Cream, half and half*					
skim, 1 cup	246	88	8.8	.2	12.5
skim, partially (2% nonfat solids), 1 cup ..	246	145	10.3	4.9	14.8
Milk, dry:					
whole, spooned, 1 cup	121	607	31.9	33.3	46.2
whole, 1 tablespoon	7	35	1.8	1.9	2.7
nonfat, regular (1⅓ cup = 1 qt.), 1 cup	68	247	24.4	5.4	35.6

	grams	calories			
nonfat, instant (⅞ cup = 1 qt.), 1 cup	104	373	37.2	7.3	53.7
buttermilk, cultured, dried, 1 cup	120	464	41.2	6.4	60.0
Milk, goat's, whole, 1 cup	244	163	7.8	9.8	11.2
Milk, malted, dry powder, 2 heaping teaspoons	19	78	2.8	1.6	13.4
Millet, whole grain, 4 oz.	114	371	11.2	3.3	82.7
Miso, see Soybeans, fermented					
Molasses, see Syrups					
Mortadella, 4 oz.	114	359	23.2	28.5	.7
Mullet, striped, raw, meat only, 4 oz.	114	166	22.2	7.8	0
Mullet, striped, raw, whole, 1 lb.	454	351	47.1	16.6	0
Mushrooms:					
raw, untrimmed, 1 lb.	454	123	11.9	1.3	19.4
raw, sliced, 1 cup	68	19	1.8	.2	3.0
canned, with liquid, 1 cup	244	41	4.6	.2	5.9
Muskmelon, see Canteloupe; Casaba; Honeydew					
Mussels, Atlantic and Pacific:					
raw, in shell, 1 lb.	454	153	22.2	3.2	7.2
raw, meat only, 4 oz.	114	108	16.3	2.5	3.8
canned, drained, 4 oz.	114	130	20.7	3.8	1.7
Mustard, prepared, brown, 1 teaspoon	10	9	.6	.6	.5
Mustard, prepared, yellow, 1 teaspoon	10	8	.5	.4	.6
Mustard greens:					
raw, untrimmed, 1 lb.	454	98	9.5	1.6	17.8
fresh, boiled, drained, 1 cup	221	51	4.9	.9	8.8
frozen, chopped, boiled, drained, 1 cup	214	43	4.7	.9	6.6

Food and measure	gram weight	calories	protein grams	fat grams	carbo-hydrate grams
Mustard spinach, boiled, drained, 4 oz. ··········	114	18	1.9	.2	3.2
Mustard spinach, raw, 1 lb. ··············	454	100	10.0	1.4	17.7
Nectarines, fresh:					
whole, 1 lb. ···········	454	267	2.5	trace	71.4
pitted, 4 oz. ···········	114	73	.7	trace	19.4
1 average ···········	50	30	.3	trace	7.9
New Zealand spinach, boiled, drained, 4 oz. ··	114	15	1.9	.2	2.4
New Zealand spinach, raw, 1 lb. ··········	454	86	10.0	1.4	14.1
Noodles, egg, cooked, 1 cup ···········	160	200	6.6	2.4	37.3
Noodles, egg, dry, 4 oz. ···········	114	440	14.5	5.2	81.6
Noodles, fried, chow-mein type, canned, 2 oz. ···	57	277	7.5	13.3	32.9
Noodles, fried, chow-mein type, canned, 1 cup	45	220	5.9	10.6	26.1
Nuts, see individual listings					
Oat or oatmeal, see *Cereals*					
Ocean perch:					
Atlantic, raw, whole, 1 lb. ···········	454	124	25.3	1.7	0
Atlantic, raw, meat only, 4 oz. ·········	114	100	20.4	1.4	0
Pacific, raw, whole, 1 lb. ···········	454	116	23.3	1.8	0
Pacific, raw, meat only, 4 oz. ·········	114	108	21.6	1.7	0
Octopus, raw, 4 oz. ···········	114	83	17.4	.9	0

Oil, cooking or salad, 1 cup	210	1856	0	210.0	0
Oil, cooking or salad, 1 tablespoon	14	124	0	14.0	0
Okra:					
raw, whole, 1 lb.	454	140	9.4	1.2	29.6
raw, fully trimmed, 4 oz.	114	41	2.7	.3	8.6
fresh, boiled, drained, slices, 1 cup	160	46	3.2	.5	9.6
fresh, boiled, drained, whole, 1 cup	177	51	3.5	.5	10.6
frozen, cuts, cooked, drained, 1 cup	184	70	4.0	.2	16.2
frozen, whole, boiled, drained, 1 cup	138	52	3.0	.1	12.1
Olive oil, see *Oil, cooking or salad*					
Olives, pickled, canned or bottled:					
green, 2 oz.	57	66	.8	7.3	.8
green, 3 extra large	16	15	.2	2.0	.2
ripe, Ascolano, Manzanilla, 2 oz.	57	73	.6	7.9	1.5
ripe, Mission, 2 oz.	57	105	.7	11.5	1.8
ripe, Mission, 2 large	10	15	.1	2.0	.3
ripe, Sevillano, 2 oz.	57	53	.6	5.4	1.5
ripe, salt-cured, oil-coated, Greek type, 2 oz.	57	193	1.2	20.4	4.9
Onions, dehydrated flakes, 1 cup	64	224	5.6	.8	5.3
Onions, green (immature), fresh:					
raw, untrimmed, 1 lb.	454	76	1.8	.3	17.6
raw, with tops, 4 oz.	114	41	1.7	.2	9.3
raw, bulb and white stem, 6 small	50	23	.6	.1	5.3
raw, slices, 1 cup	100	45	1.1	.2	10.5
Onions, mature, fresh:					
raw, untrimmed, 1 lb.	454	157	6.2	.4	35.9

Food and measure	gram weight	calories	protein grams	fat grams	carbohydrate grams
raw, 1 average (2½" diameter)	110	40	1.6	.1	9.6
raw, chopped, 1 cup	173	66	2.6	.2	15.1
raw, grated, 1 cup	231	88	3.5	.2	20.1
raw, slices, 1 cup	113	43	1.7	.1	9.8
large, boiled, drained, halves, 1 cup	179	52	2.1	.2	11.6
large, boiled, drained, whole, 1 cup	209	60	2.5	.2	13.6
pearl, boiled, drained, whole, 1 cup	185	54	2.2	.2	12.0
Onions, Welsh, raw, fully trimmed, 4 oz. ..	114	39	2.2	.5	7.4
Onions, Welsh, raw, untrimmed, 1 lb.	454	100	5.6	1.2	19.2
Orange-apricot juice drink, canned, 6 oz. glass ..	188	94	.6	.2	23.9
Orange-cranberry relish, see *Cranberry-orange relish*					
Orange-grapefruit juice:					
canned, sweetened, 6 oz. glass	185	93	.9	.2	22.6
canned, unsweetened, 6 oz. glass	185	79	1.1	.4	18.7
frozen, unsweetened, diluted, 6 oz. glass ..	175	77	1.0	.2	18.4
Orange juice:					
fresh, California navel, 6 oz. glass	186	89	1.9	.2	21.0
fresh, California Valencia, 6 oz. glass	186	87	1.9	.6	19.5
fresh, Florida, early and midseason, 6 oz. gls.	185	74	.9	.4	17.2
fresh, Florida Valencia, 6 oz. glass	186	84	1.1	.4	19.5
fresh, Temple, 6 oz. glass	186	100	.9	.4	24.0

canned, sweetened, 6 oz. glass	186	97	1.3	.4	22.7
canned, unsweetened, 6 oz. glass	186	89	1.5	.4	20.8
canned concentrate, unsweetened, 1 tablespoon	20	45	.8	.3	10.1
frozen, unsweetened, diluted, 6 oz. glass	186	84	1.3	.2	19.9
dehydrated, crystals, 1 tablespoon	8	30	.4	.1	7.1
dehydrated, diluted, prepared, 6 oz. glass	186	85	1.1	.4	20.1
Orange peel, candied, 1 oz.	28	90	.1	.1	22.8
Orange peel, fresh, 1 oz.	28	n.a.	.4	.1	7.1
Oranges, fresh:					
California navel, whole, 1 lb.	454	157	4.0	.3	39.2
California navel, 1 average (2⅗" diameter)	180	60	2.0	.2	16.0
California Valencia, whole, 1 lb.	454	174	4.1	1.0	42.2
California Valencia, flesh only, 4 oz.	114	58	1.4	.3	14.1
Florida, all varieties, whole, 1 lb.	454	158	2.3	.7	40.3
Florida, 1 average (3" diameter)	210	75	1.5	.4	19.0
segments, 1 cup	195	94	2.0	.4	23.6
Oyster stew, see *Soup, frozen*					
Oysters:					
Eastern, raw, in shell, 1 lb.	454	30	3.8	.8	1.5
Eastern, raw, meat only, 4 oz.	114	75	9.6	2.0	3.9
Eastern, raw, meat only, 1 cup (13–19 medium)	240	158	20.2	4.3	8.2
Pacific and Western, raw, meat only, 4 oz.	114	103	12.1	2.5	7.3
canned, meat with liquid, 4 oz.	114	87	9.7	2.5	5.6
frozen, meat with liquid, 4 oz.	114	n.a.	6.9	n.a.	n.a.

Food and measure	gram weight	calories	protein grams	fat grams	carbo-hydrate grams
Pancakes, prepared from mix, 4" diameter cake:					
plain, made with milk	45	91	2.7	2.5	14.4
plain, made with eggs and milk	45	101	3.2	3.3	14.6
buckwheat, made with egg and milk	45	90	3.1	4.1	10.7
buttermilk, made with milk	45	91	2.7	2.5	14.4
buttermilk, made with egg and milk	45	101	3.2	3.3	14.6
Pancreas, raw:					
beef, fat, 4 oz.	114	358	14.5	32.9	0
beef, medium fat, 4 oz.	114	321	15.3	28.4	0
beef, lean only, 4 oz.	114	160	20.0	8.3	0
calf, 4 oz.	114	183	21.8	10.0	0
hog (hog sweetbread), 4 oz.	114	274	16.7	22.6	0
Papaw, fresh, flesh only, 4 oz.	114	96	5.9	1.0	19.1
Papaw, fresh, whole, 1 lb.	454	289	17.7	3.1	57.2
Parsley, fresh, chopped, 1 tablespoon	4	2	.1	trace	.3
Parsley, fresh whole, 1 lb.	454	200	16.3	2.7	38.6
Parsnips, fresh:					
raw, whole, 1 lb.	454	293	6.6	1.9	67.5
raw, pared, 4 oz.	114	86	1.9	.6	19.8
boiled, drained, cuts, 1 cup	211	139	3.2	1.1	31.4
Passionfruit, fresh, flesh only, 4 oz.	114	102	2.5	.8	24.0
Passionfruit, fresh, whole (in shell), 1 lb	454	212	5.2	1.7	50.0

Pastina, dry:

Food					
carrot, 2 oz.	57	210	6.7	.9	42.9
egg, 2 oz.	57	217	7.3	2.3	40.7
spinach, 2 oz.	57	209	7.0	.9	42.4
Pâté de foie gras, canned, 1 oz.	28	131	3.2	12.4	1.4
Pâté de foie gras, canned, 1 tablespoon	14	65	1.6	6.1	.7
Peach nectar, canned, 6 oz. glass	185	89	.4	trace	22.9
Peaches:					
fresh, whole, 1 lb.	454	131	2.1	.3	33.4
fresh, 1 average (2" diameter)	114	35	.7	.1	10.0
fresh, diced, 1 cup	266	101	1.6	.3	25.8
fresh, slices, 1 cup	177	67	1.1	.2	17.2
canned, water pack, 1 cup	245	76	1.0	.2	20.0
canned, juice pack, 2 halves; 2 tablespoon juice	100	45	.6	.1	11.6
canned in heavy syrup, halves, 1 cup	255	199	1.0	.3	51.3
canned in heavy syrup, slices, 1 cup	253	197	1.0	.3	50.9
canned, juice pack, 2 halves; 2 tablespoons syrup	115	90	.5	.1	23.1
dehydrated, uncooked, 4 oz.	114	386	5.4	1.0	99.7
dehydrated, uncooked, halves, 1 cup	176	598	8.4	1.6	154.9
dehydrated, cooked, sweetened, with liquid, 1 cup	242	293	2.7	.5	75.7
dried, uncooked, 4 oz.	114	297	3.5	.8	77.5
dried, cooked, sweetened, with liquid, 1 cup	280	333	2.5	.6	86.2
dried, cooked, unsweetened, with liquid, 1 cup	260	213	2.6	.5	55.6

Food and measure	gram weight	calories	protein grams	fat grams	carbo-hydrate grams
frozen, sweetened, sliced, 8 oz. package	227	200	9.1	.2	51.3
frozen, sweetened, slices, 1 cup	250	220	1.0	.3	56.5
Peanut butter, 1 tablespoon	14	82	3.5	7.1	2.6
Peanut flour, defatted, 4 oz.	114	421	54.3	10.4	35.7
Peanut spread, 1 tablespoon	14	84	2.8	7.3	3.1
Peanuts:					
raw, in shell, 1 lb.	454	1868	86.1	157.3	61.6
raw, shelled, 4 oz.	114	640	29.5	53.9	21.1
roasted, in shell, 1 lb.	454	1769	79.6	148.0	62.6
roasted, shelled, 4 oz.	114	660	29.7	55.2	23.4
roasted, shelled, halves, 1 cup	144	842	37.4	71.7	27.0
roasted, shelled, chopped, 1 cup	138	807	35.9	68.7	25.9
roasted, chopped, 1 tablespoon	9	53	2.3	4.5	1.7
Pear nectar, canned, 6 oz. glass	185	96	.6	.4	24.4
Pears:					
fresh, whole, 1 lb.	454	252	2.9	1.7	63.2
fresh, 1 average (2½" diameter)	182	101	1.2	.7	25.2
fresh, slices, 1 cup	164	100	1.1	.7	25.1
canned, water pack, 1 cup	244	78	.5	.5	20.3
canned in heavy syrup, halves, 1 cup	230	175	.5	.5	45.1
canned in heavy syrup, slices, 1 cup	255	194	.5	.5	38.0
dried, uncooked, 4 oz.	114	305	3.5	2.0	76.7

	Grams	Calories	Protein	Fat	Carbohydrate
dried, cooked, sweetened, 1 cup	280	422	3.6	2.2	106.4
dried, cooked, unsweetened, 1 cup	265	328	3.8	2.0	82.4
candied, 1 oz.	28	86	.4	.2	21.5
Peas, blackeye, see *Cowpeas*					
Peas, green, immature:					
raw, in pods, 1 lb.	454	145	10.9	.7	24.8
raw, shelled, 4 oz.	114	95	7.2	.5	16.3
raw, shelled, 1 cup	138	116	8.7	.6	19.9
fresh, boiled, drained, 1 cup	163	116	8.8	.7	19.7
early or June, canned with liquid, 1 cup	250	165	8.8	.8	31.3
early or June, canned, drained, 1 cup	172	151	8.1	.7	28.9
sweet, canned with liquid, 1 cup	250	143	8.5	.8	26.0
sweet, canned, drained, 1 cup	172	138	7.9	.7	25.8
frozen, uncooked, 1 cup	145	106	7.8	.4	18.6
frozen, boiled, drained, 1 cup	167	114	8.5	.5	19.7
Peas, mature, dry:					
whole, 1 lb.	454	1542	109.3	5.9	273.5
split, without seed coat, 1 lb.	454	1579	109.8	4.5	284.4
split, cooked, drained, 1 cup	194	223	15.5	.6	40.4
Peas and carrots, frozen, boiled, drained, 1 cup	174	92	5.6	.5	17.6
Pecans:					
in shell, 1 lb.	454	1652	22.1	171.2	35.1
shelled, 4 oz.	114	779	10.4	80.8	16.6
shelled, halves, 1 cup	108	742	9.9	76.9	15.8
shelled, chopped, 1 cup	105	721	9.7	74.8	15.3
shelled, chopped, 1 tablespoon	7	48	.6	5.0	1.0

Food and measure	gram weight	calories	protein grams	fat grams	carbo-hydrate grams
Peppers, hot, chili:					
green, raw, whole, 1 lb.	454	123	4.3	.7	30.1
green, raw, seeded, 4 oz.	114	42	1.5	.2	10.3
green, pods, canned with liquid, 4 oz.	114	28	1.0	.1	6.9
red, raw, whole, 1 lb.	454	405	16.1	10.0	78.8
red, raw, pods with seeds, 4 oz.	114	105	4.2	2.6	20.5
red, raw, pods, seeded, 4 oz.	114	74	2.6	.5	17.9
red, chili sauce, canned, 1 oz.	28	6	.3	.2	.1
red, dried, pods, 1 oz.	28	91	3.6	2.6	7.4
red, dried pods, 1 tablespoon	8	26	1.0	.7	4.8
red, dried, powder, see *Chili powder*					
Peppers, sweet, fresh:					
green, whole, 1 lb.	454	82	4.5	.7	17.9
green, seeded, cored, 4 oz.	114	25	1.4	.2	5.4
green, raw, 1 average	62	14	.7	.1	3.0
green, raw, chopped, 1 cup	150	33	1.8	.3	7.2
green, raw, slices, 1 cup	82	18	1.0	.2	3.9
green, raw, strips, 1 cup	98	22	1.2	.2	4.7
green, boiled, drained, 1 average	62	11	.6	.1	2.4
green, boiled, drained, strips, 1 cup	135	24	1.4	.3	5.1
red, whole, 1 lb.	454	112	5.1	1.1	25.8
red, seeded, cored, 4 oz.	114	35	1.6	.3	8.1

	60	19	.8	.2	4.3
red, 1 average					
red, canned, see *Pimientos*					
Perch, ocean, see *Ocean perch*					
Perch, raw:					
white, whole, 1 lb.	454	193	31.5	6.5	0
white, meat only, 4 oz.	114	134	21.9	4.5	0
yellow, whole, 1 lb.	454	161	34.5	1.6	0
yellow, meat only, 4 oz.	114	103	22.1	1.0	0
Persimmons, fresh:					
Japanese or kaki, with seeds, 1 lb. ..	454	286	2.6	1.5	73.3
Japanese or kaki, seedless, whole, 1 lb.	454	293	2.7	1.5	75.1
Japanese or kaki, seedless, 4 oz.	114	87	.8	.5	22.3
native, whole, 1 lb.	454	472	3.0	1.5	124.6
native, flesh only, 4 oz.	114	144	.9	.5	38.0
Pheasant, raw, ready-to-cook, whole, 1 lb. ..	454	596	95.9	20.5	0
Pheasant, raw, meat only, 4 oz. ...	114	184	26.8	7.7	0
Pickerel, chain, raw, whole, 1 lb. ..	454	194	43.3	1.2	0
Pickerel, chain, raw, meat only, 4 oz. ..	114	95	21.2	.6	0
Pickle relish:					
sour, 4 oz.	114	22	.8	1.0	3.1
sour, 1 tablespoon	15	3	.1	.1	.4
sweet, 4 oz.	114	132	1.7	1.0	30.6
sweet, 1 tablespoon	15	21	.1	.1	5.1
Pickles, chow-chow (with cauliflower):					
sour, 4 oz.	114	33	1.6	1.5	4.7
sweet, 4 oz.	114	132	1.7	1.0	30.6

Food and measure	gram weight	calories	protein grams	fat grams	carbo- hydrate grams
Pickles, cucumber:					
dill, 8 oz.	227	25	1.6	.5	5.0
dill, 1 average (4" long)	133	15	.9	.3	2.9
fresh, bread and butter, 8 oz. ...	227	166	2.1	.5	40.6
fresh, bread and butter, 12 medium slices ..	100	73	.9	.2	17.9
sour, 8 oz.	227	23	1.2	.5	4.6
sour, 1 average (4" long)	133	13	.7	.3	2.6
sweet, 8 oz.	227	331	1.6	1.9	82.8
sweet, 1 average (2¾" long)	20	29	.1	.1	7.3
sweet, chopped, ½ cup	124	181	.9	.5	45.3
Pie crust, baked from mix with water, 9" shell	135	675	8.2	45.1	59.1
Pies, coconut custard, baked from mix, 2 oz. ..	57	116	2.5	4.5	16.6
Pies, frozen, baked:					
apple, 2 oz. slice	57	145	1.1	5.8	22.8
cherry, 2 oz. slice	57	166	1.2	6.8	25.3
coconut custard, 2 oz. slice	57	142	3.4	6.8	16.8
Pigeonpeas, dry, 4 oz.	114	388	23.1	1.6	72.2
Pigeonpeas, raw, immature seeds, in pods, 1 lb.	454	207	12.7	1.1	37.7
Pignolia, see *Pine nuts*					
Pig's feet, pickled, 4 oz.	114	227	19.0	16.9	0
Pimientos, canned, with liquid, 4 oz.	114	31	1.0	.6	6.6
Pimientos, canned, 1 average	38	10	.3	.2	2.2

Pineapple:				
fresh, whole, 1 lb.	454	123	.9	.5	32.3
fresh, diced, 1 cup	140	73	.6	.3	19.2
canned, water pack, 4 oz.	114	44	.4	.1	11.6
canned, juice pack, 4 oz.	114	66	.5	.1	17.1
canned, juice pack, 1 slice, 2 tablespoons juice	122	71	.5	.1	18.4
canned in heavy syrup, crushed, 1 cup	262	194	.8	.3	50.8
canned in heavy syrup, slices, 1 cup	278	200	.8	.3	53.9
canned in heavy syrup, 1 slice, 2 tablespoons syrup	122	90	.4	.1	23.7
canned in heavy syrup, tidbits, 1 cup	258	191	.8	.3	50.1
frozen, sweetened, chunks, 1 cup	230	196	1.0	.2	51.0
candied, 1 oz.	28	90	.2	.1	22.7
Pineapple-grapefruit juice drink, canned, 6 oz. glass	185	100	.4	trace	25.2
Pineapple juice, unsweetened:					
canned, 6 oz. glass	185	102	.7	.2	25.0
frozen, diluted, 6 oz. glass	185	96	.7	trace	23.7
Pineapple-orange juice drink, canned, 6 oz. glass	185	100	.4	.2	25.0
Pine nuts:					
pignolias, shelled, 4 oz.	114	629	35.4	54.0	13.2
pinon, in shell, 1 lb.	454	1671	34.2	159.2	53.9
pinon, shelled, 4 oz.	114	724	14.8	68.9	23.4
Pistachio nuts:					
in shell, 1 lb.	454	1347	43.8	121.8	43.1
shelled, 4 oz.	114	674	21.9	60.9	21.5

Food and measure	gram weight	calories	protein grams	fat grams	carbohydrate grams
shelled, 1 cup	125	743	24.1	67.1	23.8
shelled, chopped, 1 tablespoon	9	53	1.7	4.8	1.7
Pizza, with cheese, frozen, baked, 4 oz.	114	279	10.8	8.1	40.4
Plantain, see *Bananas, baking-type*					
Plums:					
fresh, damson, whole, 1 lb.	454	272	2.1	trace	73.5
fresh, damson, 1 average (2" diameter)	60	36	.3	trace	9.7
fresh, red, hybrid, whole, 1 lb.	454	205	2.1	.9	52.4
fresh, red, hybrid, 1 average (2" diameter)	60	27	.3	.1	6.9
fresh, red, hybrid, pitted, diced, 1 cup	164	79	.8	.3	20.2
fresh, red, hybrid, pitted, halves, 1 cup	176	84	.9	.4	21.6
fresh, red, hybrid, pitted, slices, 1 cup	169	81	.8	.3	20.8
fresh, prune-type, whole, 1 lb.	454	320	3.4	.9	84.0
fresh, prune-type, pitted, 4 oz.	114	85	.9	.2	22.3
canned, purple, water pack, 4 oz.	114	50	.4	.2	12.9
canned, purple, in heavy syrup, 1 cup	234	194	.9	.2	50.5
canned, greengage, water pack, 4 oz.	114	36	.4	.1	9.4
Poke shoots (pokeberry), boiled, drained, 4 oz.	114	23	2.6	.5	3.5
Poke shoots (pokeberry), raw, 1 lb.	454	104	11.8	1.8	16.8
Pomegranate, fresh, pulp only, 4 oz.	114	71	.6	.3	18.6
Pomegranate, fresh, whole, 1 lb.	454	160	1.3	.8	41.7
Pompano, raw, meat only, 4 oz.	114	188	21.3	10.8	0

	Grams	Calories			
Pompano, raw, whole, 1 lb.	454	422	47.8	24.1	0
Popcorn:					
unpopped, 1 oz.	28	103	3.4	1.3	20.4
popped, plain, 1 cup	11	43	1.4	.6	8.4
popped, with oil or butter, 1 cup	14	64	1.4	3.1	8.3
popped, sugar-coated, 1 cup	18	69	1.1	.6	15.4
Porgy, raw, meat only, 4 oz.	114	127	21.6	3.9	0
Porgy, raw, whole, 1 lb.	454	208	35.3	6.3	0
Pork, cured, see *Ham*					
Pork, fresh, medium-fat class:					
chop, broiled, lean and fat, 4 oz. with bone	114	297	18.6	23.6	0
chop, broiled, lean only, 4 oz. with bone	114	148	16.8	8.4	0
roast, Boston butt, cooked, lean and fat, 4 oz.	114	403	25.7	32.6	0
roast, Boston butt, cooked, lean only, 4 oz.	114	279	30.8	16.3	0
roast, loin, cooked, lean and fat, 4 oz.	114	414	28.0	32.6	0
roast, loin, cooked, lean only, 4 oz.	114	290	33.6	16.2	0
Potato chips, 2 oz.	57	324	3.0	22.7	28.5
Potato sticks, 2 oz.	57	310	3.6	20.7	28.9
Potatoes, sweet:					
raw, whole, 1 lb.	454	419	6.2	1.5	96.6
baked, 1 average	110	155	2.3	.5	35.7
boiled, 1 average	110	125	1.9	.5	28.9
boiled, drained, mashed, 1 cup	253	288	4.3	1.0	66.5
boiled, drained, slices, 1 cup	158	181	2.7	.6	41.8
candied, 1 average (3½ × 2¼")	175	294	2.3	5.8	59.9
canned, vacuum or solid pack, 1 cup	218	235	4.4	.4	54.3

Food and measure	gram weight	calories	protein grams	fat grams	carbohydrate grams
dehydrated flakes, dry, 1 cup	116	439	4.9	.7	104.4
dehydrated flakes, prepared with water, 1 cup	253	240	2.5	.3	57.2
Potatoes, white:					
raw, whole, 1 lb.	454	279	7.7	.4	62.8
raw, 1 small	100	76	2.1	.1	17.1
baked, with skin, 1 small	100	93	2.6	.1	21.1
boiled, with skin, 1 small	100	76	2.1	.1	17.1
boiled, peeled, 1 small	100	65	1.9	.1	14.5
peeled, boiled, drained, diced, 1 cup ...	156	101	3.0	.2	22.6
peeled, boiled, drained, mashed, 1 cup ...	207	135	3.9	.2	30.0
peeled, boiled, drained, riced, 1 cup ...	227	148	4.3	.2	32.9
peeled, boiled, drained, slices, 1 cup ...	159	103	3.0	.2	23.1
canned, with liquid, 8 oz.	227	100	2.5	.5	22.2
dry, see *Potatoes, white, dehydrated*					
French-fried, 10 pieces (2" long)	57	156	2.4	7.5	20.5
frozen, French-fried, heated, 17 pieces ...	85	187	3.0	7.1	28.6
frozen, hash browned, heated, 1 cup ...	200	448	4.0	23.0	58.0
frozen, mashed, heated, 1 cup	200	186	3.6	5.6	31.4
Potatoes, white, dehydrated, 1 cup:					
flakes, dry	46	167	3.3	.3	38.6
flakes, meshed with water, milk, butter	200	186	3.8	6.4	29.0

granules, dry	200	704	16.6	1.2	160.8
granules, mashed with water, milk, butter ..	200	196	4.0	7.2	28.8
Poultry, see individual listings					
Pretzels, 2 oz.	57	222	5.6	2.6	43.3
Pretzels, 3-ring, small (7 per oz.)	4	16	.4	.2	3.0
Prickly pears, raw, flesh only, 4 oz.	114	48	.6	.1	12.4
Prickly pears, raw, whole, 1 lb.	454	84	1.0	.2	21.8
Prune juice, canned or bottled, 6 oz. glass	192	148	.8	.2	36.5
Prunes:					
dehydrated, nugget type, pitted, 4 oz.	114	390	3.8	.6	103.5
dehydrated, pitted, cooked, sweetened, 1 cup ..	251	452	3.0	.5	118.2
dried, "softenized," with pits, 4 oz.	114	246	2.0	.6	65.0
dried, with pits, cooked, sweetened, 1 cup ..	258	444	2.1	.5	116.4
dried, with pits, cooked, unsweetened, 1 cup	258	307	2.6	.8	81.0
Pudding, starch base mix:					
chocolate, cooked with milk, 1 cup	290	360	9.8	8.8	66.1
chocolate, no-cook, made with milk, 1 cup ..	300	376	9.0	7.4	73.2
Pudding, vegetable gum base:					
custard, cooked with milk, 1 cup	290	380	9.0	10.2	65.6
Pumpkin:					
fresh, whole, 1 lb.	454	83	3.2	.3	20.6
fresh, pulp only, 4 oz.	114	30	1.1	.1	7.4
canned, 8 oz.	227	75	2.3	.7	17.9
canned, 1 cup	243	80	2.4	.7	19.2
Pumpkin seed kernels, dry, 4 oz.	114	630	33.0	53.2	17.0
Purslane leaves, with stems, raw, 1 lb.	454	95	7.7	1.8	17.2

Food and measure	gram weight	calories	protein grams	fat grams	carbohydrate grams
Purslane leaves, with stems, 4 oz.	114	24	1.9	.5	4.3
Purslane leaves, boiled, drained, 1 cup	180	27	2.2	.6	5.0
Quail, raw, meat and skin, 4 oz.	114	195	28.8	7.9	0
Quail, raw, ready to cook, 1 lb.	454	686	102.1	27.8	0
Quinces, fresh, flesh only, 4 oz.	114	65	.5	.1	17.4
Quinces, raw, whole, 1 lb.	454	158	1.1	.3	42.3
Rabbit:					
domestic, raw, ready to cook, 1 lb.	454	581	75.0	29.0	0
domestic, raw, meat only, 4 oz.	114	184	23.8	9.1	0
domestic, stewed, 4 oz.	114	245	33.2	11.5	0
wild, raw, ready to cook, 1 lb.	454	490	76.0	18.0	0
wild, raw, meat only, 4 oz.	114	153	23.8	5.7	0
Radishes, fresh:					
common, with tops, 1 lb.	454	49	2.9	.3	10.3
common, without tops, 4 oz.	114	17	1.0	.1	3.7
common, 4 small	40	7	.4	trace	1.4
common, whole, 1 cup	132	22	1.3	.1	4.8
common, slices, 1 cup	114	19	1.1	.1	4.1
Oriental, with tops, 1 lb.	454	57	2.7	.3	12.6

	gm	cal			
Oriental, without tops, 4 oz.	114	17	.8	.1	3.7
Oriental, pared, 4 oz.	114	22	1.0	.1	4.8
Raisins, natural:					
uncooked, 1 lb.	454	1311	11.3	.9	351.1
uncooked, 1 cup	143	413	3.6	.3	110.7
uncooked, chopped, 1 cup	162	468	4.1	.3	125.4
uncooked, ground, 1 cup	269	777	6.7	.5	208.2
cooked, sweetened, with liquid, 1 cup	243	517	2.9	.2	137.0
Raspberries:					
black, fresh, untrimmed, 1 lb.	454	321	6.6	6.2	69.1
black, fresh, 1 cup	123	90	1.8	1.7	19.3
black, canned, unsweetened, with liquid, 8 oz.	227	116	2.5	2.5	24.3
red, fresh, untrimmed, 1 lb.	454	251	5.3	2.2	59.8
red, fresh, 1 cup	140	80	1.7	.7	19.0
red, canned, unsweetened, with liquid, 8 oz.	227	79	1.6	.2	20.0
red, frozen, sweetened, 8 oz.	227	222	1.6	.5	55.8
red, frozen, sweetened, 1 cup	249	244	1.6	.5	61.3
Red snapper, see *Snapper, red and gray*					
Rhubarb:					
raw, without leaves, whole, 1 lb.	454	62	2.3	.4	14.4
raw, trimmed, 4 oz.	114	18	.7	.1	4.2
cooked, sweetened, with liquid, 1 cup	240	338	1.2	.2	86.4
frozen, sweetened, 1 cup	220	165	1.3	.4	40.7
frozen, sweetened, boiled, 1 cup	248	355	1.2	.4	89.8
Rice:					
brown, cooked, 1 cup	168	200	4.2	1.0	42.8

Food and measure	gram weight	calories	protein grams	fat grams	carbo-hydrate grams
white, long-grain, cooked, 1 cup ·········	169	179	3.5	.2	39.4
white, precooked, ready to serve, 1 cup ····	140	153	3.1	trace	33.9
Rice bran, 4 oz. ····	114	313	15.1	17.9	57.6
Rice cereal, see *Cereals*					
Rice polish, 4 oz. ············	114	301	13.7	14.5	65.4
Rolls, mix, made with water, baked, 2 oz. ····	57	170	5.1	2.6	31.1
Rolls and buns, packaged, ready to serve:					
brown and serve, browned, 2 oz. ········	57	187	4.9	4.4	31.2
hard, 2 oz. ·············	57	178	5.6	1.8	33.9
plain (pan rolls), 2 oz. ·············	57	170	4.7	3.2	30.2
raisin, 2 oz. ·············	57	157	3.9	1.6	32.1
sweet, 2 oz. ·············	57	180	4.8	5.2	28.1
whole wheat, 2 oz. ··········	57	146	5.7	1.6	29.8
Romaine, see *Lettuce*					
Rutabagas:					
raw, without tops, whole, 1 lb. ··········	454	177	4.2	.4	42.4
raw, flesh only, 4 oz. ·············	114	52	1.2	.1	12.5
raw, diced, 1 cup ·············	139	64	1.5	.1	15.3
boiled, drained, diced, 1 cup ·············	171	60	1.5	.2	14.0
boiled, drained, mashed, 1 cup ·············	243	85	2.2	.2	19.9

Sabelfish, raw, whole, 1 lb.	454	362	24.8	28.4	0
Sablefish, raw, meat only, 4 oz.	114	216	14.8	16.9	0
Safflower oil, see *Oil, cooking or salad*					
Safflower seed kernels, dry, hulled, 4 oz.	114	698	21.7	67.5	14.1
Safflower seed kernels, dry, in hull, 4 oz.	114	356	11.1	34.4	7.2
Safflower seed meal, partially defatted, 4 oz.	114	403	44.9	9.3	41.4
Salad dressings, bottled:					
blue cheese, ¼ cup	62	312	3.0	32.4	4.6
blue cheese, 1 tablespoon	15	76	.7	7.8	1.1
cooked (mayonnaise type), ¼ cup	58	252	.6	24.5	8.4
cooked (mayonnaise type), 1 tablespoon	15	65	.2	6.3	2.2
French, ¼ cup	62	254	.4	24.1	10.9
French, 1 tablespoon	15	62	.1	5.8	2.6
Italian, ¼ cup	58	320	.1	34.8	4.0
Italian, 1 tablespoon	15	83	trace	9.0	1.0
mayonnaise, ¼ cup	55	395	.6	43.9	1.2
mayonnaise, 1 tablespoon	15	108	.2	12.0	.3
Roquefort cheese, ¼ cup	62	312	3.0	32.4	4.6
Roquefort cheese, 1 tablespoon	15	76	1.0	7.8	1.1
Russian, ¼ cup	62	306	1.0	31.5	6.4
Russian, 1 tablespoon	15	74	.2	7.6	1.6
Thousand Island, ¼ cup	63	316	.5	31.6	9.7
Thousand Island, 1 tablespoon	15	75	.1	7.5	2.3
Salami, cooked, 4 oz.	114	354	19.9	29.2	1.6
Salami, dry, 4 oz.	114	513	27.1	43.4	1.4

Food and measure	gram weight	calories	protein grams	fat grams	carbo-hydrate grams
Salmon:					
Atlantic, raw, whole, 1 lb.	454	640	66.3	39.5	0
Atlantic, raw, meat only, 4 oz.	114	246	25.5	15.2	0
Atlantic, canned, with liquid, 4 oz. ..	114	232	24.8	13.9	0
Chinook or king, raw, steak, 1 lb.	454	886	76.2	62.3	0
Chinook or king, raw, meat only, 4 oz.	114	252	21.7	17.7	0
Chinook or king, canned, with liquid, 4 oz. ..	114	240	22.4	16.0	0
Chum, canned, with liquid, 4 oz.	114	159	24.5	5.9	0
Coho, canned, with liquid, 4 oz.	114	175	23.8	8.1	0
pink or humpback, raw, steak, 1 lb. ...	454	475	79.8	14.8	0
pink or humpback, raw, meat only, 4 oz. ..	114	135	22.7	4.2	0
pink or humpback, canned, with liquid, 4 oz. ..	114	161	23.4	6.7	0
red or sockeye, canned with liquid, 4 oz. ..	114	195	23.2	10.6	0
Salmon, smoked, 4 oz.	114	200	24.6	10.6	0
Salt, table, 1 lb.	454	0	0	0	0
Salt pork, raw, with skin, 4 oz.	114	853	4.2	92.5	0
Sand dab, raw, meat only, 4 oz.	114	89	18.9	.9	0
Sand dab, raw, whole, 1 lb.	454	118	25.0	1.2	0
Sandwich spread, with chopped pickle, 1 table-spoon	15	57	trace	5.4	2.4
Sapotes, fresh, flesh only, 4 oz.	114	142	2.0	.7	35.8
Sapotes, raw, whole, 1 lb.	454	431	6.2	2.1	108.9

Sardines:					
Atlantic, canned in oil, with liquid, 4 oz.	114	353	23.4	27.7	.7
Atlantic, canned in oil, drained, 3 oz.	85	173	20.4	9.4	n.a.
Pacific, raw, meat only, 4 oz.	114	182	21.8	9.8	0
Pacific, canned with mustard, 3½ oz.	100	196	18.8	12.0	1.7
Pacific, canned with brine or tomato sauce, 3½ oz.	100	197	18.7	12.2	1.7
Sauce, see individual listings					
Sauerkraut, canned, with liquid, 4 oz.	114	20	1.1	.2	4.6
Sauerkraut juice, canned, ½ cup	114	11	.8	trace	2.6
Sauger, raw, whole, 1 lb.	454	133	28.4	1.3	0
Sauger, raw, meat only, 4 oz.	114	95	20.3	.9	0
Sausage (see also individual listings):					
blood, 4 oz.	114	449	16.1	42.1	.3
brown-and-serve, browned, 4 oz.	114	481	18.8	43.1	3.2
country style, smoked, 4 oz.	114	393	17.2	35.4	0
Polish style, 4 oz.	114	346	17.9	29.4	1.4
pork and beef, chopped, 4 oz.	114	383	17.8	34.1	0
pork, links or bulk, cooked, 4 oz.	114	543	20.6	50.4	trace
pork, canned, drained, 4 oz.	114	434	20.9	37.4	2.2
scrapple, 4 oz.	114	245	10.0	15.5	16.6
Vienna, canned, 4 oz.	114	274	16.0	22.6	.3
Scallions, see *Onions, green*					
Scallops, bay and sea:					
raw, meat (muscle) only, 4 oz.	114	92	17.4	.2	3.8

Food and measure	gram weight	calories	protein grams	fat grams	carbohydrate grams
fresh, steamed, 4 oz.	114	128	26.4	1.6	n.a.
frozen, breaded, fried, reheated, 4 oz.	114	221	20.5	9.6	12.0
Scup, see *Porgy*					
Sesame seeds, dry, hulled, 4 oz.	114	660	20.7	60.6	20.0
Sesame seeds, dry, whole, 4 oz.	114	639	21.1	55.7	24.5
Shad:					
raw, whole, 1 lb.	454	370	40.5	21.8	0
raw, meat only, 4 oz.	114	193	21.1	11.4	0
canned, with liquid, 4 oz.	114	172	19.2	10.0	0
Shad roe, broiled with butter, lemon juice, 4 oz.	114	143	24.9	3.2	1.9
Shad roe, raw, 4 oz.	114	147	27.7	2.6	1.7
Shallots, fresh, peeled, 1 oz.	28	20	.7	trace	4.8
Shallots, fresh, with skin, 4 oz.	114	72	2.5	.1	16.8
Sherbet, orange, 1 cup	170	228	1.5	2.0	52.4
Shrimp:					
raw, whole, in shell, 1 lb.	454	285	56.7	2.5	4.7
raw, shelled and cleaned, 4 oz.	114	103	20.5	.9	1.7
fresh, breaded, French-fried, 4 oz.	114	255	23.0	12.2	11.3
canned, with liquid, 4 oz.	114	91	18.4	.9	.9
canned, dry pack or drained, 4 oz.	114	132	27.4	1.2	.8
frozen, raw, breaded, 4 oz.	114	158	13.9	.8	22.6
Shrimp paste, canned, 1 oz.	28	51	5.9	2.7	.4

Skate, raw, meat only, 4 oz.	114	111	24.3	.8	0
Smelt, Atlantic, jack and bay:					
raw, whole, 1 lb.	454	244	46.4	5.2	0
raw, meat only, 4 oz.	114	111	21.1	2.4	0
canned, with liquid, 4 oz.	114	227	20.9	15.3	0
Snail, giant African, raw, 4 oz.	114	83	11.2	1.6	5.0
Snail, raw, 4 oz.	114	102	18.3	1.6	2.3
Snapper, red and gray, raw, meat only, 4 oz.	114	106	22.5	1.0	0
Snapper, red and gray, raw, whole, 1 lb.	454	219	46.7	2.1	0
Soft drinks, carbonated:					
club soda, 8 oz. glass	245	0	0	0	0
cola, 8 oz. glass	245	96	0	0	24.5
cream soda, 8 oz. glass	245	105	0	0	26.9
fruit-flavor soda, 8 oz. glass	245	113	0	0	29.4
ginger ale, 8 oz. glass	245	76	0	0	19.6
quinine water (tonic), 8 oz. glass	245	76	0	0	19.6
root beer, 8 oz. glass	245	100	0	0	25.7
Sole, raw, fillets, 4 oz.	114	89	18.9	.9	0
Sole, raw, whole, 1 lb.	454	118	25.0	1.2	0
Soup, canned, condensed, diluted with equal amount of water or whole milk, 1 cup:					
asparagus, cream of, diluted with milk	238	143	6.7	5.7	16.2
asparagus, cream of, diluted with water	238	64	2.4	1.7	10.0
bean, with pork, diluted with water	249	167	8.0	5.7	21.7
beef broth, bouillon or consommé, with water	238	31	5.0	0	2.6
beef noodle, diluted with water	238	67	3.8	2.6	6.9

Food and measure	gram weight	calories	protein grams	fat grams	carbohydrate grams
celery, cream of, diluted with milk	238	164	6.2	9.0	14.8
celery, cream of, diluted with water	238	86	1.7	5.0	8.8
chicken, cream of, diluted with water	238	93	2.9	5.7	7.9
chicken, cream of, diluted with milk	238	174	7.1	10.0	14.0
chicken consommé, diluted with water	238	21	3.3	trace	1.9
chicken gumbo, diluted with water	238	55	3.1	1.4	7.4
chicken noodle, diluted with water	238	62	3.3	1.9	7.9
chicken with rice, diluted with water	238	48	3.1	1.2	5.7
chicken vegetable, diluted with water	240	74	4.1	2.4	9.4
clam chowder, Manhattan, diluted with water	240	79	2.2	2.4	12.0
minestrona, diluted with water	240	103	4.8	3.4	13.9
mushroom, cream of, diluted with milk	238	209	6.7	13.8	15.7
mushroom, cream of, diluted with water	238	133	2.4	9.5	10.0
onion, diluted with water	238	64	5.2	2.4	5.2
pea, green, diluted with milk	245	208	10.3	6.4	28.7
pea, green, diluted with water	245	130	5.6	2.2	22.5
pea, split, diluted with water	240	142	8.4	3.1	20.2
tomato, diluted with milk	240	166	6.2	6.7	21.6
tomato, diluted with water	240	86	1.9	2.4	15.4
turkey noodle, diluted with water	238	79	4.3	2.9	8.3
vegetable beef, diluted with water	240	77	5.0	2.2	9.4

vegetable with beef broth, diluted with water	240	77	2.6	1.7	13.2
vegetarian vegetable, diluted with water	240	77	2.2	1.9	13.0

Soup, frozen, condensed, diluted with equal part water or whole milk, 1 cup:

clam chowder, New England, diluted with milk	235	202	8.7	11.8	15.7
clam chowder, New England, diluted with water	235	127	4.2	7.5	10.3
oyster stew, diluted with milk	235	197	9.9	11.5	13.9
oyster stew, diluted with water	235	120	5.4	7.5	8.0
pea, green, with ham, diluted with water	235	134	8.9	2.8	18.8
potato, cream of, diluted with milk	235	179	7.5	9.2	17.6
potato, cream of, diluted with water	235	103	3.3	5.2	11.5
shrimp, cream of, diluted with milk	235	233	8.9	15.7	14.6
shrimp, cream of, diluted with water	235	155	4.7	11.8	8.2
vegetable with beef, diluted with water	235	82	6.3	2.8	8.0

Soup, mix, dehydrated:

beef noodle, dry form, 1 oz.	28	110	3.9	2.1	18.5
chicken noodle, dry form, 1 oz.	28	109	4.1	2.8	16.5
chicken rice, dry form, 1 oz.	28	100	2.6	1.9	17.8
onion, dry form, 1 oz.	28	99	3.9	3.0	15.3
pea, green, dry form, 1 oz.	28	103	6.4	1.2	17.5
tomato vegetable with noodles, dry form, 1 oz.	28	99	2.5	2.3	17.8

Soy sauce, 1 tablespoon	14	9	.8	.2	1.2
Soybean curd or tofu, 4 oz.	114	82	8.9	4.8	2.7

Food and measure	gram weight	calories	protein grams	fat grams	carbo- hydrate grams
Soybean flour, see *Flour*					
Soybean milk, fluid, 4 oz.	114	37	3.9	1.7	2.5
Soybean milk, powder, 4 oz.	114	486	47.4	23.0	31.8
Soybean protein, 4 oz.	114	365	84.9	.1	17.1
Soybean proteinate, 4 oz.	114	354	91.4	.1	8.7
Soybean sprouts, see *Bean sprouts*					
Soybeans:					
young seeds, raw, in pods, 1 lb.	454	322	26.2	12.3	31.7
young seeds, raw, shelled, 4 oz.	114	152	12.4	5.8	15.0
young seeds, boiled, drained, 4 oz.	114	134	11.1	5.8	11.5
young seeds, canned, with liquid, 4 oz.	114	85	7.4	3.6	7.2
mature seeds, dry, raw, 4 oz.	114	457	38.7	20.1	38.0
mature seeds, dry, cooked, 4 oz.	114	147	12.5	6.5	12.2
fermented (natto), 4 oz.	114	190	19.2	8.4	13.1
fermented, with cereal (miso), 4 oz.	114	194	11.9	5.2	26.7
Spaghetti:					
cooked firm, 8–10 minutes, 1 cup	130	192	6.5	.7	39.1
cooked tender, 14–20 minutes, 1 cup	140	155	4.8	.6	32.2
canned in tomato sauce with cheese, 8 oz.	227	172	5.0	1.4	34.9
canned with meatballs, tomato sauce, 8 oz.	227	234	11.1	9.3	25.9
Spinach:					
raw, trimmed (packaged), 1 lb.	454	118	14.5	1.4	19.5

raw, chopped, 1 cup	52	14	1.7	.2	2.2
raw, whole leaves, 1 cup	33	9	1.1	.1	1.4
boiled, drained, 1 cup	156	36	4.7	.5	5.6
canned, drained solids, 1 cup	223	54	6.0	1.3	8.0
frozen, leaf, boiled, drained, 1 cup	188	45	5.5	.6	7.3
frozen, chopped, boiled, drained, 1 cup ...:	188	43	5.6	.6	7.0
Spinach, New Zealand, see *New Zealand spinach*					
Spiny lobster, see *Crayfish*					
Squab (pigeon), raw, meat only, 4 oz.	114	161	19.8	8.5	0
Squash, summer:					
white, scallop, raw, whole, 1 lb.	454	93	4.0	.4	22.7
white, scallop, boiled, drained, mashed, 1 cup	238	38	1.7	.2	9.0
yellow, crookneck, raw, whole, 1 lb.	454	89	5.3	.9	19.1
yellow, crookneck, boiled, drained, diced, 1 cup	205	31	2.0	.4	6.4
yellow, boiled, drained, slices, 1 cup	176	26	1.8	.4	5.5
yellow, frozen, boiled, drained, 8 oz.	227	48	3.2	.3	10.7
zucchini, raw, whole, 1 lb.	454	73	5.2	.4	15.5
zucchini, boiled, drained, slices, 1 cup	152	18	1.5	.2	3.8
Squash, winter:					
acorn, raw, whole, 1 lb.	454	152	5.2	.3	38.6
acorn, baked, mashed, 1 cup	205	113	3.9	.2	28.7
acorn, boiled, drained, mashed, 1 cup	231	79	2.5	.7	21.3
butternut, raw, whole, 1 lb.	454	171	4.4	.3	44.4
butternut, baked, mashed, 1 cup	205	139	3.7	.2	35.9
frozen, heated, 8 oz.	227	86	2.7	.7	20.9

Food and measure	gram weight	calories	protein grams	fat grams	carbohydrate grams
hubbard, raw, whole, 1 lb.	454	117	4.2	.9	28.1
hubbard, baked, mashed, 1 cup	205	102	3.7	.8	24.0
hubbard, boiled, drained, mashed, 1 cup	235	71	2.6	.7	16.2
Squash seed kernels, dry, 4 oz.	114	630	33.0	53.2	17.0
Squid, raw, meat only, 4 oz.	114	95	18.6	1.0	1.7
Strawberries:					
fresh, whole, with caps and stems, 1 lb.	454	161	3.0	2.2	36.6
fresh, whole, capped, 1 cup	144	53	1.0	.7	12.1
frozen, sweetened, sliced, 8 oz.	227	247	1.2	.5	63.1
frozen, sweetened, whole, 8 oz.	227	209	.9	.5	53.3
Sturgeon:					
raw, meat only, 4 oz.	114	107	20.5	2.2	0
cooked, steamed, 4 oz.	114	181	28.8	6.5	0
smoked, 4 oz.	114	169	35.4	2.1	0
Succotash, frozen, boiled, drained, 1 cup	192	179	8.1	.8	39.4
Sucker, carp, raw, meat only, 4 oz.	114	126	21.8	3.6	0
Sucker, carp, raw, whole, 1 lb.	454	196	34.0	5.7	0
Suckers, white and mullet, raw, fillets, 4 oz. ..	114	118	23.4	2.1	0
Suckers, white and mullet, raw, whole, 1 lb. ..	454	203	40.2	3.5	0
Suet (beef kidney fat), 4 oz.	114	969	1.7	106.5	0
Sugar, beet or cane:					
brown, 1 lb.	454	1692	0	0	437.3

	grams	calories	protein	fat	carbohydrate
brown, firm-packed, 1 cup	212	791	0	0	204.4
brown, firm-packed, 1 tablespoon	14	52	0	0	13.5
granulated, 1 lb.	454	1746	0	0	451.3
granulated, 1 cup	195	751	0	0	194.0
granulated, 1 tablespoon	12	46	0	0	12.0
granulated, 1 lump (1⅛ × ¾ × ⅜")	6	25	0	0	6.0
powdered (confectioner's), 1 lb.	454	1746	0	0	451.3
powdered, unsifted, 1 cup	123	474	0	0	122.4
powdered, sifted, 1 cup	95	366	0	0	94.5
powdered, stirred, 1 tablespoon	8	31	0	0	8.0
Sugar, maple, 1 lb.	454	1579	n.a.	n.a.	408.0
Sugar, maple, 1 oz.	28	99	n.a.	n.a.	25.5
Sugar apple, fresh, flesh only, 4 oz.	114	107	2.0	.3	26.9
Sugar apple, fresh, whole, 1 lb.	454	192	3.7	.6	48.4
Sunflower seeds, hulled, 4 oz.	114	635	27.2	53.7	22.6
Sunflower seeds, in hull, 1 lb.	454	1372	58.8	115.8	48.7
Sweetbreads:					
beef, raw, 4 oz.	114	235	16.6	18.2	0
beef, braised, 4 oz.	114	363	29.4	26.3	0
calf, raw, 4 oz.	114	107	20.2	2.3	0
calf, braised, 4 oz.	114	191	37.0	3.6	0
hog, see Pancreas					
lamb, raw, 4 oz.	114	107	16.0	4.3	0
lamb, braised, 4 oz.	114	198	31.9	6.9	0

Food and measure	gram weight	calories	protein grams	fat grams	carbo-hydrate grams
Sweet potato, see *Potato, sweet*					
Sweetsop, see *Sugar apple*					
Swordfish, canned, with liquid, 4 oz.	114	116	19.9	3.4	0
Swordfish, raw, meat only, 4 oz.	114	134	21.8	4.5	0
Syrups (see also individual listings):					
cane, 1 tablespoon	20	53	0	0	13.6
maple, 1 tablespoon	20	50	0	0	13.0
sorghum, 1 tablespoon	20	51	n.a.	n.a.	13.6
table blend, chiefy corn, 1 tablespoon	20	58	0	0	15.0
table blend, cane and maple, 1 tablespoon ..	20	50	0	0	13.0
Tamarind, fresh, flesh only, 4 oz.	114	271	3.2	.7	70.9
Tamarind, fresh, whole, 1 lb.	454	520	6.1	1.3	136.1
Tangelo juice, fresh, 6 oz. glass	186	76	.9	.2	18.0
Tangerine juice:					
fresh, 6 oz. glass	186	80	.9	.4	18.8
canned, sweetened, 6 oz. glass	186	93	.9	.3	22.3
canned, unsweetened, 6 oz. glass	186	80	.9	.3	19.0
frozen, sweetened, diluted, 6 oz. glass	170	78	.9	.3	18.4
Tangerines:					
fresh, whole, 1 lb.	454	154	2.7	.7	38.9

fresh, whole, 1 average (2½" diameter)	114	39	.7	.2	9.7
fresh, sections only, 1 cup	193	89	1.5	.4	22.4
Tapioca, dry, 1 tablespoon	10	35	.1	trace	8.6
Taro, fresh:					
corms and tubers, whole, 1 lb.	454	373	7.2	.8	90.3
corms and tubers, without skin, 4 oz.	114	111	2.2	.2	26.9
leaves and stems, 4 oz.	114	45	3.4	.9	8.4
Tartare sauce, 1 tablespoon	14	74	.2	8.1	.6
Tea, instant, 1 teaspoon	4	1	n.a.	trace	.4
Thuringer, 4 oz.	114	348	21.1	27.8	1.8
Tilefish:					
raw, whole, 1 lb.	454	183	40.5	1.2	0
raw, meat only, 4 oz.	114	90	19.9	.6	0
baked, meat only, 4 oz.	114	156	27.8	4.2	0
Tofu, see Soybean curd					
Tomato catsup, see Catsup and Chili sauce					
Tomato juice, canned, 6 oz. glass	181	34	1.6	.2	7.8
Tomato juice cocktail, canned, 6 oz. glass	181	38	1.3	.2	9.1
Tomato paste, canned, 8 oz.	227	186	7.7	.9	42.2
Tomato paste, canned, 1 cup	258	212	8.8	1.0	48.0
Tomato puree, canned, 8 oz.	227	89	3.9	.5	20.2
Tomato puree, canned, 1 cup	250	98	4.2	.5	22.3
Tomatoes, green, fresh, whole, 1 lb.	454	99	5.0	.9	21.3
Tomatoes, ripe:					
fresh, whole, 1 lb.	454	100	5.0	.9	21.3
fresh, whole, 1 small (2½" diameter)	150	33	1.6	.3	7.0

Food and measure	gram weight	calories	protein grams	fat grams	carbohydrate grams
fresh, slices, 1 cup	181	40	2.0	.4	8.5
fresh, boiled, with liquid, 1 cup	242	62	3.2	.4	13.4
canned, with liquid, 8 oz.	227	48	2.3	.5	9.8
canned, with liquid, 1 cup	240	50	2.4	.5	10.3
Tongue, canned or cured (beef, lamb, etc.):					
whole, canned or pickled, 4 oz.	114	303	21.9	23.0	.3
potted or deviled, 4 oz.	114	329	21.1	26.1	.8
Tongue, fresh:					
beef, fat, raw, 4 oz.	114	262	17.8	20.4	.5
beef, medium fat, raw, 4 oz.	114	235	18.6	17.0	.5
beef, medium fat, braised, 4 oz.	114	277	24.4	18.9	.5
beef, smoked, 4 oz.	114	n.a.	19.5	32.7	n.a.
calf, raw, 4 oz.	114	147	21.0	6.0	1.0
calf, braised, 4 oz.	114	181	27.1	6.8	1.1
hog, raw, 4 oz.	114	244	19.1	17.7	.6
hog, braised, 4 oz.	114	287	24.9	19.7	.6
lamb, raw, 4 oz.	114	226	15.8	17.4	.6
lamb, braised, 4 oz.	114	288	23.2	20.6	.6
sheep, raw, 4 oz.	114	301	15.5	24.7	2.7
sheep, braised, 4 oz.	114	366	22.5	28.7	2.7
Tripe, beef, commercial, 4 oz.	114	113	21.7	2.3	0
Tripe, beef, pickled, 4 oz.	114	70	13.4	1.5	0

	Grams	Calories			
Trout, brook, raw, meat only, 4 oz.	114	115	21.8	2.4	0
Trout, brook, raw, whole, 1 lb.	454	224	42.7	4.7	0
Trout, lake, see *Lake Trout*					
Trout, rainbow, canned, 4 oz.	114	237	23.4	15.2	0
Trout, rainbow, raw, meat and skin, 4 oz.	114	221	24.4	12.9	0
Tuna, bluefin, raw, meat only, 4 oz.	114	165	28.6	4.7	0
Tuna, canned:					
canned, in oil, with liquid, 4 oz.	114	327	27.5	23.3	0
canned, in oil, drained, 4 oz.	114	223	27.8	7.9	0
canned in water, with liquid, 4 oz.	114	144	31.8	.9	0
Tuna, yellowfin, raw, meat only, 4 oz.	114	151	28.0	3.4	0
Turkey, canned, boned, 4 oz.	114	231	23.9	14.3	0
Turkey, fresh:					
dark meat only, roasted, 4 oz.	114	232	34.3	9.5	0
light meat only, roasted, 4 oz.	114	201	37.6	4.4	0
meat and skin, roasted, 4 oz.	114	253	36.2	10.9	0
skin only, roasted, 2 oz.	57	256	9.6	23.8	0
meat only, roasted, chopped, 1 cup	141	268	44.4	8.6	0
meat only, roasted, diced, 1 cup	135	257	42.5	8.2	0
Turkey, potted, 4 oz.	114	283	9.9	21.9	0
Turkey pot pie, frozen, 8 oz. pie	227	447	13.2	23.6	45.6
Turnip greens:					
fresh, untrimmed, 1 lb.	454	107	11.4	1.1	19.0
fresh, trimmed, 4 oz.	114	32	3.4	.4	5.7
boiled, little water, short time, drained, 1 cup	148	30	3.3	.3	5.3

Food and measure	gram weight	calories	protein grams	fat grams	carbo- hydrate grams
boiled, large amount water, long time, drained, 1 cup	148	28	3.3	.3	4.9
canned, with liquid, 1 cup	226	41	3.4	.7	7.2
frozen, boiled, drained, 1 cup	163	37	4.1	.5	6.4
Turnips:					
fresh, raw, without tops, untrimmed, 1 lb.	454	117	3.9	.8	25.7
fresh, raw, slices, 1 cup	127	36	3.8	.4	6.4
boiled, drained, diced, 1 cup	157	31	3.5	.3	5.4
boiled, drained, mashed, 1 cup	228	45	5.0	.5	7.7
Turtle, green, canned, 4 oz.	114	120	26.5	.8	0
Turtle, green, raw, meat only, 4 oz.	114	101	22.5	.6	0
Veal, fresh, meat only:					
flank, stewed, lean and fat, 4 oz.	114	446	27.2	36.9	0
foreshank, stewed, lean and fat, 4 oz.	114	245	32.5	11.8	0
loin, chop, broiled, lean and fat, 4 oz.	114	267	30.2	15.3	0
plate, stewed, lean and fat, 4 oz.	114	344	29.6	24.0	0
rib, roasted, lean and fat, 4 oz.	114	305	30.8	19.2	0
round with rump, broiled, lean and fat, 4 oz.	114	245	30.7	12.6	0
Vegetable juice cocktail, canned, 6 oz. glass	181	31	1.6	.2	6.5
Vegetable oil, see *Oil, cooking or salad*					

	grams				
Vegetables, see individual listings					
Vegetables, mixed, frozen, 8 oz.	227	148	7.5	.7	31.1
Vegetables, mixed, frozen, boiled, drained, 1 cup	182	116	5.8	.5	24.4
Venison, raw, meat only, 4 oz.	114	143	23.8	4.5	0
Vinegar:					
cider, 1 cup	239	33	trace	0	14.1
cider, 1 tablespoon	15	2	trace	0	.9
distilled, 1 cup	239	29	n.a.	n.a.	12.0
distilled, 1 tablespoon	15	2	n.a.	n.a.	.8
Waffles:					
frozen, 4 oz.	114	287	8.1	7.0	47.6
frozen, 1 double waffle	50	127	3.6	3.1	21.0
mix, dry form, 1 oz.	28	101	2.4	.5	21.5
Walnuts:					
black, in shell, 1 lb.	454	627	20.5	59.2	14.8
black, shelled, 4 oz.	114	712	23.3	67.3	16.8
black, shelled, chopped, 1 cup	119	747	24.4	70.6	17.6
black, shelled, chopped, 1 tablespoon	8	50	1.6	4.7	1.2
English, in shell, 1 lb.	454	1329	30.2	130.6	32.2
English, shelled, 4 oz.	114	738	16.8	72.6	17.9
English, shelled, chopped, 1 cup	119	775	17.6	76.2	18.8
English, shelled, chopped, 1 tablespoon	8	52	1.2	5.1	1.3
Water chestnuts, Chinese, raw, peeled, 4 oz.	114	90	1.6	.2	21.5
Water chestnuts, Chinese, raw, whole, 1 lb.	454	272	4.9	.7	66.4

Food and measure	gram weight	calories	protein grams	fat grams	carbohydrate grams
Watercress, fresh:					
untrimmed, 1 lb.	454	79	9.2	1.3	12.5
trimmed, leaves and stems, 4 oz.	114	22	2.5	.3	3.4
trimmed, leaves and stems, 1 cup	33	6	.7	.1	1.0
Watermelon, fresh:					
whole, with rind, 1 lb.	454	54	1.0	.4	13.4
whole, 1 wedge (4 × 8″, approximately 2 lb.)	925	111	2.1	.8	27.2
flesh only, 4 oz.	114	29	.6	.2	7.3
flesh only, diced, 1 cup	160	42	.8	.3	10.2
Wax gourd, raw, flesh only, 4 oz.	114	16	.5	.2	3.4
Wax gourd, raw, whole, 1 lb.	454	41	1.3	.6	9.4
Weakfish, broiled, meat only, 4 oz.	114	236	27.9	12.9	0
Weakfish, raw, meat only, 4 oz.	114	137	18.7	6.4	0
Weakfish, raw, whole, 1 lb.	454	263	35.9	12.2	0
Whale, meat only, 4 oz.	114	177	23.4	8.5	0
Wheat, parboiled, see *Bulgar*					
Wheat, whole grain:					
durum, 4 oz.	114	376	14.4	2.8	79.5
hard red spring, 4 oz.	114	374	15.9	2.5	78.4
hard red winter, 4 oz.	114	374	13.9	2.0	81.3
soft red winter, 4 oz.	114	370	11.6	2.3	81.8
white, 4 oz	114	380	10.6	2.3	85.5

Food	Grams	Calories	Protein	Fat	Carbohydrate
Wheat bran, commercially milled, 4 oz.	114	242	18.2	5.2	70.2
Wheat cereal (flakes, puffed, etc.), see *Cereals*					
Wheat flour, see *Flour*					
Wheat germ, crude, commercially milled, 4 oz.	114	412	30.2	12.4	53.0
Wheat germ cereal, see *Cereals*					
Whey, dry, 4 oz.	114	396	14.6	1.3	83.4
Whey, liquid, 1 cup	244	63	2.2	.7	12.4
Whitefish, lake:					
raw, whole, 1 lb.	454	330	40.3	17.5	0
raw, meat only, 4 oz.	114	176	21.4	9.3	0
smoked, meat only, 4 oz.	114	176	23.7	8.3	0
White sauce, standard recipes:					
thin, 1 cup	250	303	9.8	21.8	18.0
medium, 1 cup	255	413	9.9	31.9	22.4
thick, 1 cup	247	489	9.9	38.5	27.2
Whiting, see *Kingfish*					
Wild rice, raw, 4 oz.	114	400	16.0	.8	85.4
Wine, see *Alcoholic beverages*					
Yam, tuber, raw, with skin, 1 lb.	454	394	8.2	.8	90.5
Yam, tuber, raw, pared, 4 oz.	114	115	2.4	.2	26.3
Yam bean, tuber, raw, pared, 4 oz.	114	62	1.6	.2	14.5
Yam bean, tuber, raw, with skin, 1 lb.	454	225	5.7	.8	52.2
Yams, canned or frozen, see *Potatoes, sweet*					

Yeast:

baker's compressed, 1 oz.	28	24	3.4	.1	3.1
baker's compressed, 1 cake	22	19	2.7	.1	2.4
baker's, dry, 1 oz.	28	80	10.5	.5	11.0
baker's, dry, 1 tablespoon or 1 package	7	20	2.6	.1	2.7
brewer's, dry, debittered, 1 oz.	28	80	11.0	.3	10.9
brewer's, dry, debittered, 1 tablespoon	8	23	3.1	.1	3.1

Yogurt:

made from partially skim milk, 8 oz. container	227	114	7.7	3.9	11.8
made from partially skim milk, 1 cup	249	125	8.5	4.2	12.9
made from whole milk, 8 oz. container	227	141	6.8	7.7	11.1
made from whole milk, 1 cup	246	153	7.4	8.4	12.1

Zucchini, see *Squash, summer*